Dinner

Desserts, Sweet Treats & Snacks 108

Sauces & Dips 122

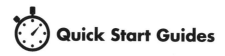

Quick Start Guides

What Can I Eat?
ON A
SUGAR FREE
DIET

A Quick Start Guide To Quitting Sugar

Lose Weight, Feel Great and Increase Your Energy!

PLUS over 100 Delicious Sugar-Free Recipes

First published in 2014 by Erin Rose Publishing

Text and illustration copyright © 2014 Erin Rose Publishing

Design: Julie Anson

ISBN: 978-0-9928232-3-8

A CIP record for this book is available from the British Library.

DISCLAIMER: This book is not intended as a substitute for the medical advice of physicians. The reader should regularly consult a physician in matters relating to his/her health and particularly with respect to any symptoms that may require treatment, diagnosis or medical attention.

Some of the recipes in this book include nuts. If you have a nut allergy it's important to avoid these. The author and publisher disclaim responsibility for any adverse effects that may result from the use or application of the recipes and information within this book.

CONTENTS

Recipes

INTRODUCTION

"If giving up sugar was so easy we'd all have done it by now! I've ditched the cakes and chocolate and I still can't lose weight!"

Those were the words of a frustrated friend in response to the latest media coverage on obesity, the modern epidemic endangering our lives. Does this sound familiar? Sure it does. She's not alone in her despair, because despite making 'healthy' changes to her diet and lifestyle, she still wasn't able to feel energetic or shift the belly bulge.

It's easy to be overwhelmed by all the information about fat, sugar and nutrition out there and not know which way to turn to improve your diet and wellbeing. It's easy to take things at face value, and believe that what we are being told is healthy is just that, but there is so much conflicting advice, it's little wonder we're confused about what to eat! It can be demoralising to try so hard and get nowhere; all the while the effects of too much sugar are keeping you trapped in a cycle of cravings and fluctuating moods. The brain fog caused by sugar makes it a struggle for basic things to make sense, the fatigue shakes your willpower, and weight gain and anxiety plummet your self-esteem, propelling you to seek comfort in food.

If you're really ready to change your life for the better then this Quick Start Guide to a Sugar-Free Diet is the perfect place to begin.

The news that not all fats are bad and that sugar can actually be far worse for our health has finally filtered through to the masses, and we're now seeking the tools to help us kick the sugar habit and make the changes that put us on the path to good health and wellbeing.

This Quick Start Guide takes a comprehensive approach to understanding sugar and its effect on your body, and provides simple steps to eliminating it for good. The idea of cutting sugar out of your life will obviously feel daunting at first, but once you take the first step forward you will quickly shift from feeling 'OK' (or maybe even feeling OK is an exaggeration) to feeling great. And the best bit is; it's YOU that makes the difference!

No more highs and lows: bursts of energy and clarity, quickly followed by lethargy, anxiety and unexplained depression. Sound familiar? Or perhaps you're just sick and tired of feeling 'sick and tired'?

This isn't just about turning down dessert or avoiding the obvious sugar traps, but it is about identifying the sneaky harmful sugars which are in so many apparently 'healthy' savoury foods. Would you really be so quick to buy those 'low-fat' yogurts if you realised that they actually contain double the amount of sugar than a regular one?

By following the guidelines in this book you can lose weight, improve your health, increase your energy levels and unleash the fitter and calmer you.

Are you ready? Let's go!

THE
SWEET
DECEIT

the Bitter Truth

Sugar affects us all in many different ways, and symptoms that you may have assumed were unrelated could actually be caused by the everyday sugar you are currently consuming.

This list isn't for medical diagnosis, but it is an indicator of the different ways fluctuating blood sugar levels could be affecting you. Before changing your diet, you should consult your doctor to find out if there is an underlying cause. If your symptoms are unexplained, it would be incredibly beneficial to take steps to cut out sugar. You don't need to be obese or even fat to be experiencing blood sugar problems. Or perhaps you are already further down the line than that. Have you already been diagnosed with diabetes?

SYMPTOM CHECKER

- Inability to lose weight
- Tiredness after eating
- Irrational when hungry
- Craving sugar, sweets and carbohydrates
- Panic attacks and unexplained anxiety
- Depression (crying spells)
- Poor memory
- Brain fog, difficulty concentrating
- Light-headedness
- Heart palpitations and tachycardia (rapid heart rate)
- Insomnia
- Shaking
- Irritability
- Desire for stimulants like caffeine, chocolate or cigarettes
- Excessive sweating
- Cold extremities and numbness
- Fatigue
- Excessive thirst
- Sudden tiredness and inability to concentrate
- Visual disturbance

The Effects Of Too Much Sugar

- Sugar is bad for the heart, even in healthy people.

- Excessive sugar consumption leads to high blood pressure and increases the risk of heart disease and strokes.

- According to an NHS Diabetes Audit, diabetics are 48% more likely to have a heart attack.

- It's responsible for increased yeast infections like thrush.

- Ferments in the gut causing wind, bloating and diarrhoea and IBS symptoms.

- It's been linked to fertility problems.

- A Netherlands university study showed higher levels of glucose lead to looking older, due to slower collagen production.

- It has been linked with dementia, as continual high blood sugar damages blood vessels and reduces oxygen to the brain.

- Recent studies suggest that those with high blood sugar are more likely to develop cancer of liver, bowel, breast and pancreas.

- It can cause fatty liver disease. If insulin is less effective, sugar gets stored as fat in the liver, and as we become less sensitive to insulin, it heightens the risk of type 2 diabetes.

- It can cause migraines and headaches due to sleep irregularities from sugar consumption.

Simplifying Blood Sugar

In basic terms, when we eat, carbohydrates are digested and absorbed as sugar which is taken up in the blood, and either used immediately or stored as glycogen. Insulin is secreted by the pancreas relative to the body's blood sugar levels to allow the glucose into the cells. Low insulin results in the diminished ability to control sugar levels, leading to high blood sugar. It's like a pendulum effect, and it's important to avoid large swings in blood sugar. A rapid rise will result in more insulin being secreted and can cause a rapid low, with some pretty unpleasant symptoms.

The pancreas and adrenals eventually become exhausted, resulting in further declining insulin levels, leading to high blood sugar and diabetes. But let's not get carried off on a negative wave here. You can get off the rollercoaster ride of spiking sugar levels. The aim is to keep it in the middle, avoid extremes and learn to relax more.

PRE-DIABETES

Pre-diabetes is often a precursor to the onset of Type 2 Diabetes. This can manifest as borderline sugar levels. If this is picked up soon enough, it can mark the turning point, and dietary and lifestyle changes can turn things around and prevent the condition from getting worse.

METABOLIC SYNDROME, AKA SYNDROME X

Another aspect of problems due to sugar is Syndrome X. This is also a risk factor for developing Type 2 diabetes. Syndrome X is characterised by tiredness, poor ability to focus, weight gain (especially around the middle) and insulin resistance. If you are concerned, your doctor can do a test to assess your blood sugar levels and advise you of your risk. Remember, diabetes develops when the body either doesn't produce sufficient insulin, or it doesn't use it effectively i.e. insulin resistance.

Insulin resistance means that instead of glucose being used by the body, it will be turned into fat – that is, until it can re-balance. There is a theory that people who over-secrete insulin, resulting in hypoglycaemia (low blood sugar) as a result of the pancreas producing too much insulin, can go on to develop Type 2 diabetes. Fluctuating highs and lows can destabilise sugar levels further, and as the pancreas becomes 'exhausted' it no longer functions in the way it should.

The symptoms of this could present as reactive hypoglycaemia, or low blood sugar episodes, occurring within four hours of a meal. With such changeable sugar levels, it could be difficult to diagnose. A prolonged glucose tolerance test, carried out by your doctor, may be helpful.

NO MORE THE CARB JUNKIE

So many of us automatically reach for a carbohydrate-rich meal or snack when we're hungry and short of time. We also associate it with comfort and use it as a stress-reliever. The feel good factor is short lived. It's a quick fix, one that picks up your blood sugar and serotonin levels, then dumps you straight after.

Once your blood sugar levels are more balanced, you won't crave this kind of stodgy food so much. Many of these recipes in this Quick Start Guide are low in carbohydrate for that reason. It's not worth making the effort to eliminate sugar, then overloading your digestion with starchy food which will turn to sugar and fat. Ditch the love affair with sugar - it wasn't working for you anyway!

DON'T UNDERESTIMATE THE EFFECT OF STRESS

The problems of excess sugar are well documented, but the warning signs that your body is already struggling with the effects of sugar may be there. Often, what is presumed to be emotional disturbances are the result of nor-mal mood fluctuations, exacerbated by sharp changes in sugar levels. Some healthcare professionals advise patients suffering with anxiety to stop all stimulants such as coffee, tea, alcohol and sugar, to help with their symptoms and help them find an even keel.

The body's natural 'fight or flight' response dramatically influences blood sugar levels, by triggering a release of adrenaline. Nowadays, our primal stress reaction is triggered by lifestyle pressures; work, financial commitments and relationships. These don't require 'flight' reaction (usually!) so the sugar levels stay high, rather than burning off energy by physical action. Chronic stress leads to fatigue and adrenal exhaustion, which worsens hypoglycaemia (low blood sugar).

A short energy blast is given by stimulants, such as coffee, tea, alcohol, chocolate, cigarettes and so-called energy drinks which are heavy with glucose. They stimulate the release of glucose into the bloodstream, causing a sharp rise in blood sugar and further stimulating the adrenals. Oh the joy!

This cycle will create cravings and a powerful desire for a quick fix which perpetuates the sharp peaks and troughs in sugar levels. Quick fixes are a temporary solution but with long-term consequences. There was a time when it was advised to just trade in pasta, white rice and bread, for brown, wholemeal alternatives. But this is not enough; especially if you are showing signs of blood sugar imbalance and particularly if you wish to lose weight. Protein helps, and there aren't many people who haven't heard of the Atkins diet. The recipes in this book take a more balanced approach which will help you get a wide variety of nutrients to nourish your body and keep you full.

The Masked Culprit - Fructose

The harmful effects of sugar are well documented. But what about our consumption of natural, and apparently healthy sugar – Fructose? Fructose consumption is one of the top reasons the 'healthy' eaters in our population have become frustrated with their results; from hunger pangs to expanding waist lines. It's become normal to have a large glass of orange juice with breakfast, and an apple juice with dinner, but this 'healthy' habit has been overwhelming us with sugar. A glass of fresh apple juice has 6 ½ teaspoons of sugar, whereas a can of fizzy drink has around a teaspoon less! Fructose is metabolised in the liver which is fine in small amounts and with the fruit's own fibre, however we consume copious amounts which are harmful and are shown to result in a fatty liver. In the case of fruit juices, most of the fibre has been removed, so you are effectively left with liquid sugar.

One expert commented that fructose should come with a health warning, similar to that of a packet of cigarettes. Seem extreme? Maybe not. Here's why.

Fructose is converted and stored as fat, rather than being used as fuel. Fruit sugar is naturally occurring and found in fruits and vegetables. Fruit is great and full of nutrients, but we need to watch the sugar content. Fructose makes us crave more and is stored in the liver, unlike glucose which is taken up by the blood stream and used immediately. That's not letting glucose off the hook, overconsumption of all sugars are responsible for the surge in obesity and bulging waist lines, but fructose is converted to fat immediately in the body.

So many of us have ditched the chocolate bars and sugary drinks and reached for apparently healthy cereal bar and a large glass of pure orange juice instead. It's frustrating when you think you're making a great effort to eat the right things and yet you're still unable to lose weight. Does this sound familiar? If you've quit the sweet treats, and been honest with yourself about how much sugar you are actually consuming, and are still unable to make progress, then fructose could be the culprit. Please remember, just because something is sold in a health shop, does not make it healthy!

*A real revelation is that **agave syrup**, which is derived from natural sugar, which has a low glycaemic index, is loaded with concentrated fructose and is actually bad for you. It's widely used as a healthy sweetening alternative.*

Let's differentiate between naturally occurring fructose in whole fruits and vegetables, and that which is processed and added to food products, such as high fructose corn syrup. Avoid anything which has been processed, cleared of all fibre and concentrated. It's highly processed. Agave syrup is very high in fructose. Depending on the brand, agave can contain anything from 75% to 92% fructose. The quantity of fructose in agave is considerably higher than high-fructose corn syrup, which is 55%. And also much higher than white table sugar, which is 50% fructose, thus making agave syrup more harmful than either high fructose corn syrup or white refined sugar.

The fact that agave syrup is high in low-glycemic fructose is often hailed as a benefit of using it. What many people don't realise is that it is concentrated fructose. Here is a startling fact; the Glycemic Index Institute of Washington DC delisted and banned it due to it being harmful to participants in studies.

For so many people who already have a healthy diet, the effect of fructose on the body has to be the biggest eye-opener. It's frustrating for so many people who've made positive changes to their diet and were unwittingly sabotaging themselves with a high intake of fruit sugar.

Artificial Sweeteners

Sweeteners, with exception of stevia which we'll get to in a minute, have created controversy since the 1970's, and have been linked with cancers, a higher BMI and lead to conflicting scientific results on the safety of chemical sweeteners, added to diet soft drinks, sweets and cough medicines.

Artificial sweeteners such as saccharin, sucralose and aspartame are completely artificial chemical sweeteners made by highly-industrial processes. None of them have calories or glycemic index, and they have been linked to cancer and chronic illnesses in numerous studies. Yet studies still produce conflicting and inconclusive results. There are still reports that they are harmful and yet they are still being added to everyday food. Sucralose is made from refined sugar which has a molecule of chlorine added to it so it isn't properly digested by the body. Aspartame also has an aftertaste which some find dislikeable. Basically, they aren't real food.

One concern about artificial sweeteners is that they affect the body's ability to gauge how much has been consumed. Some studies show that sugar and artificial sweeteners affect the brain in different ways. At the University of California, San Diego, researchers found the human brain responds to a sweet taste with signals to eat more. By providing a sweet taste without any calories, it will cause us to crave more sweet foods and drinks. Not what you need to kick the sugar habit!

Included in this book are recipes which have included the use of stevia to give you the safest option for a sweetener. Stevia or sweet leaf is derived from the South American Stevia Rebaudiana plant. It won't elevate your blood sugar and doesn't contain calories.

Fat Facts!

Fat has had a lot of bad press, but it's actually necessary to eat some fats. They are a valuable source of energy.

The clue is in the name: **Essential Fatty Acids.**

These are vital for nerves, brain, skin and forming hormones. It's not easy to over indulge with healthy fatty foods – you'll hit your 'off' switch pretty quickly – unlike sugar. Instead of hitting a sugary snack, opt for a healthy fat option.

GOOD FATS:

Coconut	Peanuts	Flaxseeds
Avocado	Sunflower seeds	Olives
Walnuts	Eggs	Oily fish (salmon, mackerel, trout and sardines)

It's the artificial trans fats you want to avoid as their chemical structure has been changed by heating and hydrogenation. They are found in margarine, fried food, factory produced cakes and biscuits. On labels, you find them listed as hydrogenated or partially hydrogenated oils or fat. And butter is better than margarine.

What Can I Eat?

DON'T EAT THESE:

Any food containing sugar: read all labels.

- Avoid all fizzy and sugary drinks, including diet drinks with artificial sweeteners such as, aspartame, xylitol, sucralose, cyclamates, saccharin, acesulfame potassium
- All dried fruit, including dates, apricots, raisins, sultanas, apples, bananas, mango, pineapple, figs etc;
- Pure or concentrated fruit juices
- Cakes, biscuits, muesli, granola, muffins, cereal bars, sweets
- Breakfast cereals (where sugar added to ingredients)
- Sucrose
- Maltose
- Dextrose
- Corn syrup
- Glucose syrup
- Fructose
- High fructose corn syrup
- Agave nectar
- Honey
- Jam
- Golden syrup
- Maple syrup
- Treacle
- Molasses
- Ready-made sauces like relish, ketchup and barbecue sauce

DO EAT THESE:

If it's green, you can go ahead.

Cooking from scratch means you know exactly what is going into your food.

Eat protein with every meal. It staves off hunger and has little effect on blood sugar. Make sure you have plenty of high protein snacks available.

- Chicken, pork, lamb, turkey, beef.
- Prawns, cod, salmon, and mackerel – oily fish are especially good.
- Uncoated nuts; Brazils, hazelnuts, cashews, peanuts and pecans
- Sunflower, sesame and pumpkin seeds.
- Cheese
- Eggs
- Yogurt
- Nut butters; peanut, almond, cashew
- Tinned tuna and sardines
- All fresh vegetables (Note; beetroot, carrots & onions are higher in fructose so reduce or avoid these if you're struggling with cravings and watching your weight.
- Raspberries, blueberries, kiwi, blackberries, rhubarb, lime, lemons
- Brown rice, quinoa, wholemeal bread (check label for sugar content)
- Popcorn
- Herbal teas (fruit teas – check sugar content)
- Reduce or remove sugar from tea and coffee
- Coconut flakes
- Corn
- Coconut oil
- Olive oil
- Cooked/sliced meats like cooked chicken, prawns or ham which you can nibble on.

Quinoa, pronounced 'keen wah' is a high protein grain which is packed with goodness, so it really is a wonder food to help break the starchy carbohydrate cravings for white bread or cakes.

Watch out for things like relishes, sauces, pickles and sun-dried tomatoes which can have sugars much higher than their fresh counterparts.

Fruit Sugars

Avoid fruit for the first 2-4 weeks. It'll help your cravings. It sounds harsh, because fruit has so many benefits, but while you're in the early stages of being sugar-free it could tickle your taste buds and tempt you to have more fruit or even sugary snacks. The body can usually tolerate a maximum of 2 pieces of fruit a day. Some of the recipes included in this book do have fruit in them and it's probably best to keep the back section with dessert recipes until you feel confident that you're in control of your sugar consumption. You don't want to come undone too early.

After that, whenever you are having fruit, make sure have it in its entirety i.e. including the fruit's fibre because the fibre it contains delays absorption of carbohydrates and sugar.

Here are the sugar contents of fruits, so you can choose how strict you wish to be. If you are insulin resistant or trying to lose weight you may wish to avoid these. And without exception, steer clear of all dried fruit.

SUGAR CONTENT OF FRUIT PER 100G

Figs	16g
Grapes	16g
Mango	14g
Pomegranate	14g
Banana	12g
Pineapple	10g
Apple	10g
Blueberries	10g
Kiwi fruit	9g
Oranges	9g
Cherries	8g
Papaya	8g
Peaches	8g
Honeydew melon	8g
Watermelon	6g
Strawberries	4.9g
Raspberries	4.4g
Lemon	2.5g
Lime	1.7g
Rhubarb	1.1g

4 g of sugar = 1 teaspoon

But let's be sensible about this and not worry too much about the numbers. Having a couple of pieces of whole fruit is nowhere near as harmful as adding refined sugars and fibre-free fructose. The nutrients are valuable and the taste sensation important to add variety to your diet, not to mention pure enjoyment. The best way to eat fruit is in its whole, natural state as the fibre will slow down the absorption. Pure fruit juices, and those from concentrate, are basically liquid fructose and will result in a higher blood sugar, pouring sugar straight into your liver and setting you up for a low afterwards. It's the swing that can create unexplained mood swings, shakiness and fatigue.

The sugar content of vegetables is generally much lower that than in fruit. Sweet tasting vegetables often thought to be high in sugar are still lower than that of most fruits. Carrots come in at 4.7g, pumpkin at 2.8g and spinach at 0.4g. However beetroot, even unsweetened, has a sugar content of 7g, almost as much as honeydew melon.

The guide is to allow you to select which fruit to choose when you reintroduce fruit into your diet. All fruit has great nutritional value, but 100g of raspberries only has a quarter of the sugar of figs, so choose wisely and you could keep your sugar intake low and still have fresh fruit daily.

ALCOHOL

With a lot of alcoholic drinks, it's the mixers which are high in sugar and are difficult if not impossible to avoid if you drink spirits. Soda is about your only option as a mixer. Gin and vodka are lower in sugar, as is dry wine. Red wine has slightly less sugar than white. Avoid desert wine, cider, and liqueurs.

How To Read The Labels

So you pick up cooked chicken in the supermarket, thinking it's just chicken, right? Wrong. Often during cooking, chicken and other meats have been basted with dextrose. Dextrose is another name for glucose, so it's best avoided. Cooked and sliced meats like Chinese or barbecue chicken that have been coated with a marinade almost certainly contain added sugar. Here are some of the alias's sugar is also known as. Avoid these.

- INVERT SUGAR SYRUP

- CANE JUICE CRYSTALS

- DEXTRIN

- DEXTROSE

- GLUCOSE SYRUP

- SUCROSE

- FRUCTOSE SYRUP

- MALTODEXTRIN

- BARLEYMALT

- BEET SUGAR

- CORN SYRUP

- DATE SUGAR

- PALM SUGAR

- MALT SYRUP

- DEHYDRATED FRUIT JUICE

- FRUIT JUICE CONCENTRATE

- CAROB SYRUP

- GOLDEN SYRUP

- REFINERS SYRUP

- ETHYLMALTOL

Be Prepared!

Take a few days to process what it is you are going to eat. Stock up on ingredients and empty your cupboards of temptations. There really is no bad time to start - the sooner the better, but if you have an upcoming party or celebration, you may want to get that under your belt before you begin.

If you haven't already, start cutting out those obviously sugar-laden foods, the fizzy drinks, sweets, cakes, chocolate. It'll make it easier when you go cold turkey!

CONSIDER TAKING SOME SUPPLEMENTS

OK, it's worth acknowledging that if your diet is well balanced, your digestion is A1 and your lifestyle is stress-free, you shouldn't need supplements. If this is you, great! However, if you're like the majority, you may need to make healthy changes to get all your nutrients. Deficiencies may need corrected. Inadequate nutrition and a busy lifestyle may have depleted your reserves.

Vitamin B

B vitamins help your body to deal with stress and it's particularly important for the nervous system, so it's helpful to get enough B vitamins when you are cutting out sugar. It's available naturally in brown rice, turkey, tuna, pulses (legumes) and bananas. A good quality, B complex will help supplement any B vitamins that are lacking.

Vitamin C

Vitamin C supports the adrenal glands, so it's really useful to combat stress as it's involved in the production of corticosteroid hormones in the adrenals, so it's a welcome boost. Yes, we do get vitamin C from fruits and vegetables, however we know that too much fruit can elevate sugar levels and you want to avoid this. Vitamin C is found in Brussels sprouts, lemons, limes, red and green peppers (bell peppers), cabbage, broccoli, cauliflower - and you won't have to worry about the sugar content. If you choose a Vitamin C supplement, avoid those with sugar or artificial sweeteners.

Magnesium

In the UK, official data showed 42% of men and 72% of women don't consume enough dietary magnesium. American research showed that people with low magnesium levels had a 94% greater chance of developing diabetes than those with the highest magnesium levels. You could do worse than take a magnesium supplement to ensure you're getting enough. It's involved in muscle relaxation, and coming off sugar can be challenging enough. Anything which helps frayed nerves and helps reduce stress has got to be good news. Dietary sources of magnesium are pumpkin seeds, lima beans, black-eyed peas, Brazil nuts, almonds, peanuts, brown rice, baked beans and shrimps.

Start Being Sugar-Free

DON'T COUNT DOWN, JUST DO IT!

As your preparation takes shape, don't set yourself a start date. It's like building a wall for you to jump over. Don't make it hard for yourself. Easy does it. Once your cupboards are re-stocked, you've had a look at some recipes and given yourself and idea of what you want to cook, taper the sugar-free changes into your lifestyle. Your target is to have as little sugar as possible.

There is still disagreement amongst experts about the maximum advisable sugar levels. But it's agreed that:

> **Your maximum daily intake should be 6-9 teaspoons a day, that's 24 – 36g.**

If something has more than 22g sugar per 100g, this is considered to be high. If it has less than 5g sugar per 100g it's considered low.

1 teaspoon = 4 grams. Be aware of this when checking the sugar content on labels.

It may seem daunting at first, but when you achieve the upper limit you can then reduce it further. Keep fruit consumption to no more than 2 pieces per day, ideally none for the first month. Keep to low sugar fruits if you wish to eat more.

When you cut out sugar, gradually implement it to get up and running. If you put too much focus on having a start date, you could find yourself thinking 'it's been 17 hours since I've had sugar' so slide into your sugar-free lifestyle. You don't need to announce to friends and family what you're doing – it may add pressure and expectation.

People are well-meaning, but talking it up will only make you think about it more. Imagine announcing to friends that you're quitting sugar and their response. They may say things like 'I could never do that' or 'I couldn't survive without my daily chocolate' or similar negative comments.

We all know sweet stuff tastes great, that's why we've been eating so much of it! So step out of the cycle of what you 'can't' do and just do it; quietly and confidently. Even if only for a few days until you get into your stride. You can tell people what you've accomplished or you could wait until they notice the difference, either in your vitality or your weight loss. Go you!

What To Expect

So let's not sugar coat this! If you've been eating what is classed today as a normal diet, you've probably been consuming too much sugar, and that's without adding it to your coffee; it's hard to avoid it. Therefore, expect some cravings. These can vary in degree, depending on what your current sugar consumption is. Your body will adjust to getting nutrients from less blatant sources, converting fuel from healthy foods which have no empty calories and are packed with goodness. So diminish any thoughts of sugary food, and do something else. Cravings? What cravings? Shrink the thoughts to noth-ing and quickly that will become you're reality. So while you are adjusting, distract yourself, think of something else, get some exercise, snack on some protein like nuts, cheese, cold meats and plenty of water. Taking a walk will keep you away from the kitchen.

How Water Can Help You

Water can really help you flush out your system, give you something to do and make you feel full, especially in between meals. Drinking plenty of water really is beneficial. It's generally accepted that 8 glasses a day is optimal. What really makes a huge difference is consuming water first thing in the morning before anything else has gone into your stomach. Why, I hear you ask? Not a coffee or a peppermint tea? Nope, clear cool water.

Large volumes of fluid leave the stomach and pass through to the intestines quicker than small volumes. Cool fluids empty more quickly too. A great way to hydrate quickly in the morning is to have a pint of cool water and add a slice of lemon if you wish. It'll break your fast and carry away the waste products your body has processed while you have slept. So, hydrate your body and start off well. You will feel bright eyed, have clearer thoughts and it will clear early morning fatigue.

How To Deal With Cravings

If sugar cravings kick in well before your next meal, apart from snacking on something high protein one of the best ways to overcome cravings is to use distraction. Literally, get up and do something. Give yourself something else to think about.

TIPS

- Exercise really helps! Get up and do something. Even gentle exercise like walking, swimming or cycling.

- Snack on protein instead of carbohydrates. Coconut chips, nuts, seeds, olives, cheese and meat.

- At mealtimes, replace starchy carbohydrates with lots of veggies and you'll feel less sluggish and hungry.

- Avoid dried fruit (it's loaded with fructose) – have nuts instead.

- Olives are a quick, easy and satisfying snack.

- Schedule in easy meals, plan in advance so you avoid temptation. That way you can also avoid missing a meal.

- Eating little and often is great. Five meals/snacks a day is best but watch your portion sizes.

- Drink plenty of water!

- Prepare some cucumber water. Steep sliced cucumber and mint leaves in a large jug of water, store in the fridge and serve with ice and lemon.

- Pamper yourself with a bath, perhaps add magnesium salts to boost your magnesium and help you relax if cravings are making your irritable.

- Prepare some tasty meals and treats for the fridge or freezer. Have something sugar-free close by so that you aren't tempted.

- Get plenty of rest and sleep.

- To avoid a mid-morning lull, start your day with a protein breakfast like eggs and bacon.

- Watch your starchy food and carbohydrate consumption, especially flour products.

- At mealtimes, replace carbohydrates with heaps of veggies. That way you won't feel so sluggish.

- Carry on-the go snacks protein like nuts, cheese, and cooked meat for quick sustenance.

- A teaspoon or two of peanut butter, straight from the jar can help you feel satisfied. Likewise for coconut oil.

- Don't criticise yourself for giving in to temptation occasionally, just carry on being sugar-free and treat it as a minor glitch. Be warned though, if you do hit the sugar you will trigger sugar cravings so you'll need to focus on getting back on track. Fats and protein can help you with that.

Detox Symptoms & Balancing Out

Sugar cravings are the simplest of the many different sugar withdrawal symptoms, which in a few cases can include headaches and lethargy. But the benefits outweigh temporary irritations. Remind yourself how well you've done. If you can manage it for one day, you can manage it for two, and if you can do it for two you can do it for a week, then another. Before you know it cravings will only be a memory. Once you start feeling better and there is more room inside your clothes, the temporary challenges will have subsided. That's when your achievement is really noticeable.

EXPERIMENTING, FEELING GOOD & MAKING IT LAST

Adding In Fruit

So now you've gotten the hang of what you can and can't eat and you have a selection of your favourite ingredients, you can play around with them. Experiment. You're bound to find your own staples which are handy and quick to prepare.

Try more of the recipes or swap tips with friends. If you've been pretty strict with yourself and avoided fruit for the first 2-4 weeks, you may want to add it into your diet now. Keep it to a maximum of 2 pieces a day. Maybe try an occasional treat. The sweet treat and chocolate recipes are included as a treat and are to be eaten in moderation. Don't overindulge. We don't want your taste buds leading you astray to similar things which are much higher in sugar. If this happens, give yourself a little longer without sweet tasting treats. At the end of a meal, snack on nuts or cheese instead.

Keep It Going! - You've Come This Far

You can stick to your sugar-free diet for a month or you can just keep on going and sugar-free can be your new normal. Treat it as a lifestyle change and your new way of eating. That's not to say you have to avoid it completely forever, it should never feel like a punishment, but once you're aware of the hidden sugars and the problems it creates you will already be way ahead and for the most part you will be sugar-free.

Simple Recipes That Make Cutting Out Sugar Easy

The recipes in this book are easy to fit into a busy schedule, simple to follow and very tasty. We don't want you to feel deprived when you give up sugar. On the contrary, reducing your sugar intake will reset your taste buds and as they adjust you'll savour the more subtle flavours in your food.

Experimenting is the key, and finding out what works for you. Once your kitchen cupboards are stocked with what you like, you can play around with the recipes and find your favourites. Get creative and make it easier for yourself, put the right kind of temptation in your way: include in your diet something which you can really look forward too. Coconut is an amazing treat ingredient - it's a sweet, satisfying, ingredient that won't play havoc with your sugar levels.

The best way to know exactly what you are eating is to make your own food from scratch. It may not take as much time as you think. When you cook from scratch, using good whole ingredients, you won't feel the need to add the unnecessary sugar which is added to the sauces of many convenience meals. To begin with you'll be re-training your taste buds to enjoy the other subtler flavours instead a sugar hit.

 Steaming a batch of squash or pumpkin, blending until smooth and storing in the freezer in an ice cube tray means it can be used in small quantities in your cooking as a secret sweet ingredient. As you adjust to being sugar-free you'll be less inclined to want the sugar hit anyway. In the early days of kicking the sugar habit, you may find it easier to have five or six small meals a day to sustain a reasonable blood sugar and prevent fluctuations while your body is adjusting to your new way of eating.

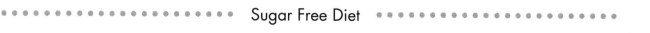

Recipes

BREAKFAST

It really is the most important meal of the day; so never miss it! Fuelling your body in the morning will kick start your energy, reviving your body and mind, to begin your day well. In Chinese Medicine, it is understood that each organ in the body has a time of high and low functioning, alternating in two hour cycles.

The stomach's peak energy time is between 7am and 9am, before the spleen energy kicks in between 9am and 11am, which helps get the nutrients from our food become utilised by the body. Even if you are fasting overnight, which is really popular and very useful for detox and weight loss, it's best to have your last meal of the day in early evening, to avoid missing breakfast completely.

Avoid a mid-morning lull and start your day with a protein breakfast like eggs and bacon. Smoothies made in a blender are a wonderfully nutritious start, but the same is not true for juices as the liquid is extracted without the fibre. Remember, we want the fibre to slow down absorption.

Smoky Baked Eggs

Ingredients

2 large eggs
30g spinach
1 teaspoon olive oil
1 garlic clove, crushed
1 teaspoon smoked paprika
1 tablespoon crème fraiche

SERVES 2

Method

Heat the oil in a pan and add the garlic and paprika. When the garlic starts to soften, add the spinach. Cook for 2-3 minutes until the spinach is wilted. Divide the spinach and the garlic between 2 ramekin dishes then break an egg into each one. Spoon half of the crème fraiche over each egg and sprinkle with smoked paprika. Place the ramekins in a preheated oven at 220C/425F for 15 minutes, until the eggs are set. Serve and enjoy.

For a variation, line the ramekin dishes with smoked salmon and top with an egg, for a rich Sunday morning treat.

Breakfast Burrito

Ingredients

4 large lettuce leaves (romaine and iceberg lettuce work best)

1 tablespoon olive oil

2 shallots, chopped

1 clove garlic, chopped

½ green pepper, chopped finely

4 eggs, beaten

1 teaspoon cumin

½ teaspoon cayenne pepper

150g (5oz) chicken (or other leftover meat)

SERVES 2

Method

Heat the oil in a frying pan, add the shallots and garlic. Cook for 5 minutes, until soft. Add the green pepper, cumin, cayenne pepper and chicken and cook for around 3 minutes. Add the eggs and scramble everything together. Serve the filling wrapped in large lettuce leaves. Without the flour tortilla, it makes a high protein breakfast which won't leave you hungry mid-morning.

Mini Meatloaves

Ingredients

8 rashers (strips of bacon)
225g (1/2 lb) bacon, chopped
450g (1lb) minced beef (ground beef)
1/2 teaspoon nutmeg
4 tablespoons chives, chopped
1 tablespoon fresh parsley, chopped
60ml (2 floz or 1/4 cup) coconut milk
2 cloves of garlic, finely chopped
Freshly ground black pepper

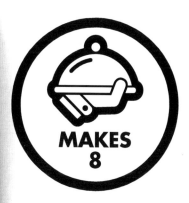

MAKES 8

Method

Preheat oven to 200C/400F. In a large bowl, combine the minced beef, bacon, garlic, nutmeg, parsley, chives and coconut milk. Mix well and season with black pepper. Use an 8-hole muffin tin, and line each hole with a strip of bacon. Spoon the beef mixture on top of the bacon. Bake the mini meatloaves in the oven for 30 minutes. Remove from the muffin tin and serve.

Tomato, Cheese & Olive Frittata

SERVES 2

Ingredients

75g (3oz or 1/2 cup) black olives
4 large eggs
8 cherry tomatoes, halved
110g (4oz or 1/2 cup) cream cheese
Sea salt
Freshly ground black pepper
1 tablespoon olive oil

Method

Cut the olives into half, removing all stones. Crack the eggs into a bowl and Whisk. Season with salt and pepper. Heat the oil in a small frying pan and pour in the egg mixture. Add in the tomatoes and olives, cut side up. Add the cream cheese, making little dollops over the top of the frittata. Cook until the mixture completely sets. Place the frittata under a hot grill for 3 minutes. The eggs should be set and the cream cheese soft. Gently remove from the pan, cut into slices and serve.

Cheese & Herb Scrambled Eggs

SERVES 2

Ingredients

4 eggs

40g (1½ oz or ½ cup) cheddar cheese, grated

1 green pepper, finely chopped

2 tablespoons fresh parsley, chopped

2 tablespoons fresh basil, chopped

1 tablespoon olive oil

Method

Put the eggs in a small bowl and whisk. Stir in the parsley and basil then set aside. Warm the oil in a frying pan, add the green pepper and sauté for 3 minutes until soft. Add the green pepper to the egg mixture. Pour the eggs into the frying pan, and stir with a spatula to scramble the eggs. Add the grated cheese and continue scrambling until the cheese has melted.

Ham & Chestnut Mushroom Omelette

Ingredients

2 eggs

1 slice of ham, chopped

2 medium-sized chestnut mushrooms, chopped

40g (1½ oz or ½ cup) cheddar cheese, grated

1 teaspoon of parsley

1 tablespoon olive oil

SERVES 1

Method

Put the eggs in a small bowl and whisk. Stir in the parsley, ham and mushrooms. Warm the oil in a small frying pan and add the egg mixture. Cook for 1 minute and allow it to start to set without stirring. Then add the grated cheese. Continue cooking until the eggs are set firm and the cheese is softened.

Boiled Egg & Asparagus Dippers

Ingredients
- 4 large eggs
- 1 bunch of asparagus
- Sea salt
- Freshly ground black pepper

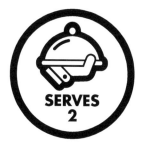

SERVES
2

Method

Place the eggs in a saucepan of boiling water and cook for 4 minutes. Meanwhile, steam the asparagus for 3 to 4 minutes, until tender. Drain the eggs and place into egg cups. Cut the tops off and serve a few spears of asparagus on a plate next to it. The asparagus can be used to dip into the runny yolks and are a great healthy alternative to toast.

Devilled Eggs

Ingredients
- 4 hard-boiled eggs, halved
- 2 tablespoons coconut oil
- 1 teaspoon ground ginger
- Paprika to season

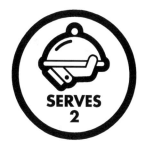

SERVES
2

Method

Remove yolks from the halved eggs and place in a small bowl. Add coconut oil and ginger then mash together with a fork. Using a teaspoon, scoop the yolk mixture back into each half of the egg. Sprinkle paprika on top.

Warm Fruit Souffle Omelette

Ingredients

1 tablespoon butter
2 eggs
100g (4oz) of raspberries,
blueberries or an apple

SERVES 1

Method

Heat the fruit in a saucepan for 5 minutes and mash with a fork until soft. Set aside. Separate the egg yolks from the white and keep the yolks in a separate bowl while you whisk the egg whites into soft peaks. Then fold the yolks into the mixture.

Heat the butter in a small frying pan and add the eggs. Cook the omelette until the eggs have set. It should be light and fluffy. Serve open on a plate, add the fruit and fold over. Serve and eat straight away. It's a lovely twist on a savoury omelette and a real family favourite.

Spinach & Apple Smoothie

Ingredients
- ½ carrot
- ½ apple
- ½ cucumber
- Handful of kale or spinach or rocket
- 1 tablespoon sunflower seeds
- 2 teaspoons sesame seeds

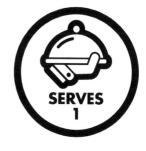

SERVES 1

Method

Place all the ingredients into a blender and around a cup of water. Blitz until smooth. You can add a little extra water if you don't want it too thick.

Blueberry & Coconut Smoothie

Ingredients
- 175ml (6fl oz) coconut milk
- ½ cup blueberries
- ½ banana
- 2 tablespoons organic plain yogurt
- 1 tablespoon coconut oil

SERVES 1

Method

Toss all the ingredients into a blender and blitz. Pour and enjoy!

Spinach & Cucumber Smoothie

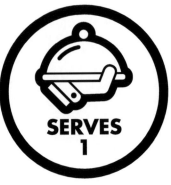

SERVES 1

Ingredients

½ cucumber
2 stalks celery
1 cup spinach leaves
1 carrot

Method

Put all the ingredients into a blender with a cup of water, and blitz until smooth. You can add ice to some blenders which can make your drinks really refreshing.

Almond Flour Pancakes

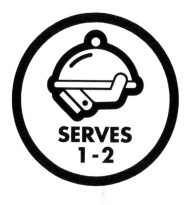

SERVES 1-2

Ingredients

2 eggs
60ml (2fl oz or 1/4 cup) water
125g (4 1/2 oz) almond flour
1 teaspoon baking powder
2 teaspoons coconut oil
Pinch of cinnamon

Method

Put the eggs in a bowl, whisk them and set aside. Combine the dry ingredients in a separate bowl and stir in the beaten eggs. Add water and mix until you have a smooth batter. Heat a little coconut oil in a frying pan. Pour a small amount of mixture into the pan to make small pancakes. Cook the pancakes until golden brown. Serve with a sprinkle of cinnamon.

Coconut Pancakes & Blueberry

Ingredients

For the pancakes:

3 eggs
90g (3 ½ oz or 1 cup) oats
2 tablespoons desiccated (shredded) coconut
1 tablespoon chia seeds
120ml (4fl oz or ½ cup) coconut milk
1 teaspoon vanilla extract
1 banana, mashed
1 teaspoon coconut oil

For the compote:
60ml (2fl oz or ¼ cup) coconut milk
1 tablespoon chia seeds
75g (½ cup) blueberries

SERVES 2

Method

Hold back the banana but combine all the other pancake ingredients in a mixing bowl. Rest the mixture for 10 minutes to allow thicken. Add the mashed banana and mix thoroughly. Heat the coconut oil in a frying pan. Spoon the pancake mixture into the pan and reduce the heat. Flip the pancakes over and cook until golden.

Add the chia seeds to the coconut milk and set aside. Warm the blueberries in a pan and crush them with a fork. Add the blueberries to the coconut milk and stir. Serve the pancakes with the blueberry compote.

High Protein Coconut & Almond Pancakes

Ingredients

2 eggs
50g (2oz or ½ cup) almond flour
50g (2oz or ½ cup) rice flour
1 tablespoon desiccated (shredded) coconut
1 teaspoon coconut oil
1 teaspoon baking powder
2 teaspoons sesame seeds

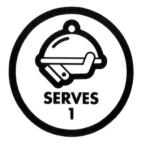

SERVES 1

Method

Whisk the eggs and set aside. Add the dry ingredients to a large bowl. Stir the whisked eggs into the dry ingredients, mixing until the batter is smooth. Heat a teaspoon of coconut oil in a frying pan. Spoon some of the mixture into the pan. Smaller pancakes work best, as being a gluten free recipe, the pancakes are very soft and light. When bubbles appear, turn them over to finish cooking.

Pancake Toppers

To keep variety in your diet, try one of the options below or experiment to find your favourite.

Banana & orange
Raspberry & blueberry
Blackberry & apple

To make the pancake toppers, simply blitz a small portion of your ingredients in a blender and pour over your pancakes. You can add a pinch of cinnamon or a squeeze of lemon juice for extra zing.

LUNCH

It can be difficult to have the time, or sometimes even the inclination to come up with something tasty and healthy for lunch, and grabbing a quick snack (eaten quickly, so mentally it doesn't really count!) is often the simplest thing to do. But don't forget, if you're short of time and imagination is lacking, by using your refrigerated leftovers you can come up with mouth watering meals you wouldn't have otherwise put together. Keep all leftovers from the night before, or even freeze them. Often throwing them into a frying pan, warming through and perhaps adding a topping of cheese or an egg can provide you with a stable and nutritious meal.

Glass mason jars with a sealed lid, are a great way of storing, and carrying salads. They are an excellent way to put together a quick, healthy meal that's easy to carry (see recipe). It takes very little preparation and they are colourful and appetising. Remember to have some protein with every meal to make sure you don't get hungry and balance your blood sugar.

Broccoli & Fennel Soup

Ingredients

2 heads of broccoli, chopped
1 fennel bulb
1 tablespoon of fresh tarragon
2 tablespoons crème fraiche (optional)
Freshly ground black pepper, to season

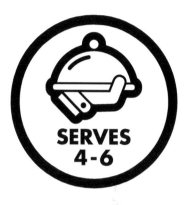

**SERVES
4-6**

Method

Place the broccoli and fennel in enough water to cover them and bring to the boil.
Simmer for 7 minutes until they are soft but tender. Add the fresh tarragon, transfer
to a food processor and blend until smooth. Add the crème fraiche and stir. Serve into
bowls and eat immediately. As a variation, you could substitute the tarragon for dill,
coriander (cilantro) or parsley.

Chicken Soup

Ingredients

225g (8oz) chicken, cut into small cubes
1 litre (1½ pints) chicken stock
1 courgette (zucchini), finely chopped
1 carrot, chopped
1 stick of celery, chopped
2 stalks of asparagus, chopped
½ teaspoon lemon juice
1 tablespoons olive oil
Sea salt
Freshly ground black pepper

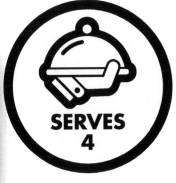

SERVES 4

Method

Heat the olive oil in a frying pan. Add the chicken and cook for 10 minutes. Place the chicken, stock and lemon juice into a large saucepan. Cook for 5 minutes. Add the courgette (zucchini), carrot, celery and asparagus. Continue cooking for around 20 minutes, until the vegetables are soft. Season the soup with salt and pepper. Serve and eat immediately.

Butternut Squash & Ginger Soup

Ingredients

1 medium onion, chopped
1 butternut squash, peeled, de-seeded and chopped
1 litre (1 ½ pts) of vegetable stock
4cm fresh root ginger, chopped
120ml (4fl oz or ½ cup) coconut milk
1 tablespoon olive oil

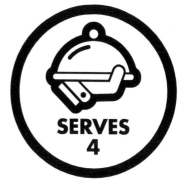

SERVES 4

Method

In a large saucepan, heat the olive oil and add the onion. Cook for 4 minutes, until the onion begins to soften. Add the squash, ginger and vegetable stock and bring to the boil. Reduce the heat and cook for 15 minutes, until the squash is soft. Pour the soup into a blender and blitz until smooth. Stir in the coconut milk. Return to the heat and warm through then serve.

Lettuce & Basil Soup

Ingredients

150g (5oz or 1 cup) potato, peel and diced
1 large onion, peel and thinly sliced
2 teaspoons olive oil
2 small round lettuce or 1 iceberg lettuce, shredded
2 tablespoons fresh basil, chopped
3 tablespoons crème fraiche
600ml (1pt) vegetable stock
Freshly ground black pepper

SERVES 4

Method

Place the oil, potato and onion in a saucepan and stir. Cover and cook on a medium heat for 8 minutes. Add the stock and bring to the boil. Season with pepper then reduce the heat and simmer for 5 minutes. Add the lettuce and simmer for another 7 minutes. Add the basil and blend the soup until smooth. Add the crème fraiche and stir. Season, sprinkle with fresh basil and serve.

Kale & Butterbean Soup

Ingredients

1 1 teaspoon olive oil
1 onion, peeled and finely chopped
1 stick celery, finely chopped
1 carrot, peeled and diced
475 ml (1pt or 2 cups) vegetable stock
150g (5oz or 1 cup) butter beans
150g (5oz or 1 cup) curly kale
1/2 teaspoon tomato puree (paste)
1/2 teaspoon oregano
1 clove garlic, crushed
Salt
Freshly ground black pepper

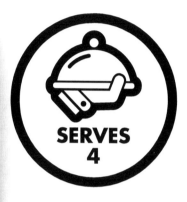

SERVES 4

Method

Heat the olive oil in a large saucepan and add the garlic, together with all of the vegetables, apart from the kale. Stir for 2 to 3 minutes on a medium heat. Add the vegetable stock and bring to the boil. Reduce the heat and cook for 15 minutes. In a food processor, blend half of the butter beans and add them to the soup. Add the kale, the remaining butter beans, tomato puree and oregano. Stir and cook for 10 minutes. Season and serve into bowls. If you prefer your soup smooth, pour it into a food processor and blend until smooth.

Mozzarella, Tomato & Basil Caprese

SERVES 4

Ingredients

4 large tomatoes
110g (4oz) mozzarella cheese
2 teaspoons olive oil
1 tablespoon basil pesto
A handful of fresh basil leaves
Freshly ground black pepper

Method

Cut the tomatoes and mozzarella into slices, around 1cm thick. Lay them out on a flat plate in a circle, alternating between slices of tomato and mozzarella. Season a little black pepper. Drizzle the basil pesto over the tomatoes and mozzarella. In the centre of the plate, place the fresh basil leaves and sprinkle with olive oil. Serve and eat immediately.

Smoked Mackerel Pate

Ingredients

2 smoked mackerel fillets, skin removed
4 tablespoons crème fraiche
1 tablespoon mayonnaise
½ teaspoon fresh dill, finely chopped
Squeeze lemon juice
Sea salt
Freshly ground black pepper

SERVES 2

Method

Place the mackerel fillets in a bowl and mash with a fork. Add the crème fraiche, mayonnaise, dill and mix together. Add a squeeze of lemon juice, with salt and pepper to season. Spoon into 2 small bowls or ramekin dishes and serve.

Vegetable Sushi Rolls

Ingredients

- 8 Nori sheets
- 150g (5 oz or 1 cup) grated carrots
- 150g (5oz or 1 cup) red pepper, finely chopped
- 150g (5oz or 1 cup) cucumber, finely chopped
- 150g (5oz or 1 cup) alfalfa sprouts
- 150g (5oz or 1 cup) brown rice
- 1 ripe avocado, chopped
- 2 teaspoons fresh dill or chives, chopped
- Tahini or hummus

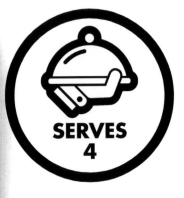

SERVES 4

Method

Lay out the nori sheets (shiny side down). Spread the tahini or hummus onto the nori sheets. Across the middle of the sheet, make a row of rice. Leave one inch of the nori sheet uncovered to seal the sushi roll. Add carrots, red pepper, cucumber, alfalfa and avocado. Top with a sprinkling of dill or chives. Season with salt and pepper. Tightly roll the nori sheet from the bottom to make a firm sushi roll. Cut into 1 inch pieces and serve. As a variation, try spreading the sushi with guacamole instead of tahini or hummus.

Crab Omelette

Ingredients

1 green chilli, seeds removed

110g (4oz or 1 cup) fresh crabmeat, cooked

2 teaspoons ginger root, finely chopped

6 spring onions, (scallions) thinly sliced

1 cup mange tout (snow peas), trimmed

4 eggs

2 teaspoons soy sauce

1 teaspoon fish sauce

1 teaspoon olive oil

SERVES
2

Method

Finely chop half of the chilli and place in a bowl with the crab, ginger and half the spring onion. Stir and set aside. Chop the remaining chilli. Place in a separate bowl with the mange tout (snow peas) and the remaining half of the spring onion (scallion). Set aside. Lightly beat the eggs, and add the soy and fish sauce. In a frying pan, heat the olive oil and pour in the egg mixture to make a flat unbroken omelette shape. Once the egg is set, transfer it to a plate. Then down the centre of the omelette, spoon the crab mixture. Roll up and slice in half. Serve topped with the mange tout and spring onions.

Halloumi
& Pancetta Rolls

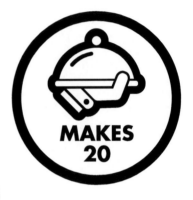

**MAKES
20**

Ingredients

10 slices of pancetta (or bacon rashers)
250g (9 oz) halloumi cheese
1 tablespoon chives, choppeds

Method

Heat the oven to 200C/400F. Cut the halloumi into 20 equal sized sticks. Sprinkle each stick with chives. Cut the slices of pancetta in half then wind a piece around each stick of halloumi to make a tight roll. Arrange on a baking sheet. Place the rolls in the oven for 10-12 minutes or until the pancetta is starting to become crispy.

Smoked Salmon Whirls

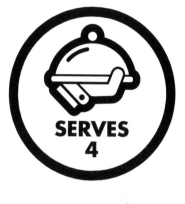

SERVES 4

Ingredients

6 slices of smoked salmon

200g (7oz) soft cream cheese

¼ teaspoon cayenne pepper

Freshly ground black pepper

1 lemon, cut into wedges

Method

Cut the salmon slices in half, lengthways. Combine the cheese, cayenne pepper and black pepper. Evenly spread the cheese mixture over the salmon. Roll up the salmon, tightly. Chill in the fridge until ready to serve. Remove the salmon rolls from the fridge, cut into slices and garnish with wedges of lemon.

Tabbouleh

SERVES 4

Ingredients

120g (4oz or 2/3 cup) quinoa, cooked

1 tomato, diced

1 cucumber, peeled and diced

75g (3oz or 1/2 cup) spring onions
(scallions), chopped

4 tablespoons fresh mint, chopped

4 tablespoons fresh parsley, chopped

1 tablespoon olive oil

Juice of 1 lemon

Sea salt

Freshly ground black pepper

Method

Combine all the ingredients in a large bowl and mix well. Cover and place in the fridge
for 20 minutes to chill or until you are ready to serve.

Cauliflower Cheese with Hazelnuts

Ingredients

SERVES
4

1 tablespoon butter

40g (1 1/2 oz or 1/4 cup) finely chopped hazelnuts

1 clove garlic, chopped

50g (2oz or 1/2 cup) grated Cheddar cheese

2 tablespoons parsley

1 cauliflower, cut into florets

Method

Heat the butter in a frying pan. Add the hazelnuts and cook for one minute until lightly toasted. Add the garlic and cook for one more minute. Remove from the heat and place in a bowl to cool. Break the cauliflower into florets and steam until tender and crisp. Place in an oven proof dish. Add the cheese and parsley to the hazelnut mixture. Cover the steamed cauliflower with the cheese and hazelnut mixture. Place under a hot grill for a few minutes until the cheese begins to bubble. Alternatively you can place in the oven to cook the cheese and keep hot until ready to serve.

Quick Curried Prawns

SERVES 6

Ingredients

24 large, prawns (shrimps), raw and peeled
2 teaspoons curry powder
2 cloves of crushed garlic
60g (2oz or ½ stick) butter for frying

Method

Melt the butter in a frying pan over a low heat. Quickly stir in the curry powder and garlic. Add the prawns. Cook for 3 to 5 minutes on each side, or until the prawns are completely pink and cooked thoroughly. Transfer them to a serving dish and pour the curry butter over them.

Smoked Mackerel and Butterbean Salad

Ingredients

- 1 tin of drained butterbeans
- 400g (14oz) trimmed green beans
- 1 small bunch of spring onions (scallions), chopped
- 2 smoked mackerel fillets, skin removed
- Lemon juice
- Freshly ground black pepper

SERVES 2

Method

Slice the runner beans and steam them for 5 minutes, or until they soften but maintain their crunch. Mix the green beans in a bowl with the butterbeans and add the chopped spring onions. Chop the 2 mackerel fillets into small pieces, and mix it all together. Season with lemon juice and serve.

Winter Salad with Macadamia Nuts

Ingredients

SERVES 2

For the dressing:

2 teaspoons olive oil
30ml (1fl oz or 1/8 cup) apple cider vinegar
1 1/2 tablespoons thyme, finely chopped
1/2 teaspoon mustard
Freshly ground black pepper

For the salad:

1 tablespoon olive oil
80g (3oz or 1/2 cup) green beans
125g (4 1/2 oz or 2/3 cup) broccoli, chopped
75g (3oz or 1/2 cup) green pepper (Bell pepper), deseeded and sliced
75g (3oz or 1/2 cup) mange tout (snow peas)
2 tomatoes, quartered and deseeded
2 spring onions (scallions), chopped
3 tablespoons roasted macadamia nuts, chopped

Method

For the dressing, combine the olive oil, vinegar, thyme and mustard in a bowl and mix well. Season with black pepper. Heat a tablespoon of olive oil in a frying pan. Add the green beans, broccoli, mange tout (snow peas) and green pepper. Stir and cook for 3 minutes. Add the tomatoes and spring onions (scallions) and heat through. Add the dressing, and coat all the vegetables. Serve into bowls and sprinkle with macadamia nuts.

Quinoa & Fresh Herb Patties

SERVES 2

Ingredients

9 0g (3 ½ oz or ½ cup) quinoa, cooked

2 eggs

2 tablespoons spring onions (scallions), chopped

2 tablespoons chopped mint

2 tablespoons chopped parsley

45g (2oz or ½ cup) grated Gruyere cheese

30g (1oz or ½ cup) fresh whole-wheat breadcrumbs

¼ teaspoon sea salt

2 teaspoons olive oil

Method

Place the eggs in a large bowl and whisk. Add onion, mint, parsley, cheese, breadcrumbs and salt. Mix well. Add the cooked quinoa and combine with the other ingredients. Heat 2 teaspoons of olive oil in a large frying pan. With clean hands, form 8 patties. Place them in the pan and cook for about 3 minutes on each side or until golden brown.

SALAD JARS

Use a glass Mason jar as a container for your favourite salad using fresh ingredients and they will keep for days. You can make them in advance at the start of the week and store them in the fridge, ready to go. These handy jars keep it fresh and transportable. Follow this principle; heavier ingredients and salad dressing goes on the bottom, the middle layers will act as a buffer and protect your lighter, delicate food such as lettuce, spinach and kale on top. Create your own combination. Mix and match these ideas and layer them up.

1 - THE BOTTOM LAYER

Basic or herb vinaigrette, garlic, basil, ginger, walnut oil, sesame oil, chilli flakes, soy sauce, olive oil, vinegar, Caesar dressing, guacamole, hummus. Mixed bean salad mix, like butterbeans, kidney beans, black eyed peas or chickpeas.

2 - THE MIDDLE LAYER

Tomatoes, grated carrots, chopped celery, spring onions, peppers, olives, bean sprouts, courgette (zucchini), radish, coleslaw, pickles, broccoli, avocado, mushrooms, rice, couscous, quinoa. Chicken, tuna, turkey, steak, mackerel, ham, crispy bacon, prawns, mozzarella, feta cheese, walnuts, sunflower seeds, cashew nuts and eggs

3 - THE TOP LAYER

Baby spinach, kale or lettuce. Fresh herbs like coriander, parsley and basil.

TACO SALAD

Use what you might want in a taco, kidney beans, chilli flakes, olive oil. Add guacamole to it. Layer tomatoes, mushrooms peppers, onions, steak or chicken. Top it off with grated cheese and lettuce.

GREEK SALAD

Start with basic vinaigrette. Layer with cucumber, tomatoes, onions, black olives, avocado. Add feta cheese cut into small cubes. Top it off with baby spinach or lettuce.

ITALIAN SALAD

Add basil vinaigrette to the bottom with a layer of butter beans. Add a layer containing olives, tomatoes, carrots, peppers, celery, onion, cucumber. Next add sliced mozzarella or cooked chicken or ham. Finish with a layer of romaine lettuce. (Avoid using sun-dried tomatoes in this one, they are much higher in sugar than fresh ones.

Sugar-Free Baked Beans

Ingredients

2 x 400g tins cannellini beans, rinsed and drained

1 x 400g tin of chopped tomatoes

1 onion, peeled and very finely chopped

1 clove garlic, crushed

1 teaspoon smoked paprika

1 large sprig rosemary

1/2 teaspoon cinnamon

1/4 teaspoon nutmeg (optional)

1 tablespoon olive oil

Splash of Worcestershire sauce

SERVES 4

Method

Heat the oil in a frying pan and add the onion, garlic and rosemary. Fry for 4 or 5 minutes, until the onion is soft. Add the smoked paprika, cinnamon and nutmeg (if desired) and stir. Add the cannellini beans and tomatoes. Reduce the heat and simmer for around 20 minutes. You may need to add a little water. Add a splash of Worcestershire sauce and season with salt and pepper. Simmer for another few minutes to reduce down. Remove the rosemary sprig and serve.

Potato Skins

Ingredients

4 large potatoes
2 tablespoons olive oil
2 teaspoons paprika
125g (4oz) pancetta, chopped
5 tablespoons crème fraiche
125g (4oz) Cheddar cheese
1 tablespoon parsley, freshly chopped

SERVES 4

Method

Preheat the oven to 200C/400F. Prick potatoes with a fork and place them on the top shelf of the oven. Bake for 1 hour or until soft right through. Leave the potatoes to cool. Cut in half and scoop the flesh into a bowl and set aside. Combine the oil and paprika and use some of it to brush the outside of the potato skins. Place under a hot grill for 5 minutes, until crisp, turning occasionally. Heat the remaining oil and paprika and fry the pancetta until it's crispy. Add this to the potato flesh, along with the crème fraiche, cheese and parsley. Mix well. Fill the potato skins with the mixture. Place the skins in the oven for a further 15 minutes, making sure they are heated thoroughly.

Quinoa, Feta & Broccoli Salad

Ingredients

300g (11oz) quinoa, cooked
200g (7oz) broccoli
200g (7oz) feta cheese, crumbled
3 tablespoons pumpkin seeds
2 tablespoons fresh mint leaves,
roughly chopped
2 tablespoons parsley, roughly chopped
3-4 tomatoes, chopped
1 bunch spring onions (scallions),
finely chopped
3 tablespoons olive oil
3 tablespoons lemon juice

SERVES 4

Method

Cut the broccoli into small bite-size pieces. Add them to a steamer and cook for 5 minutes then allow to cool. In a small frying pan, lightly toast the pumpkin seeds until they're slightly crunchy. Remove from the pan and leave to cool. Put the quinoa and broccoli in a bowl and add the feta, herbs, tomato, spring onions, pumpkin seeds, olive oil and lemon juice. Toss together until everything is mixed. Season to taste and either serve straight away or store in the fridge.

Avocado & Black Eyed Pea Salad

Ingredients

1 tablespoon lime juice

1 1/2 tablespoons olive oil

425g (15 oz) black eyed peas, drained

2 avocados, halved with stone removed

1/2 red pepper, finely chopped

1 garlic clove, minced

1/8 tsp ground paprika

1 teaspoon chopped coriander (cilantro)

Sea salt

Freshly ground black pepper

SERVES 4

Method

To make the dressing, put the lime juice in a large bowl and whisk in the olive oil. Stir in the peas, red pepper, coriander (cilantro), garlic, paprika, salt and black pepper. Mix together until everything is coated with the dressing. Place the avocado halves on 4 plates. Spoon the mixture over the avocado and serve.

Feta & Courgette Cakes

Ingredients

1 courgette (zucchini)
120g (4oz or 1 cup) butter beans, rinsed
50g (2oz or 1cup) feta cheese, crumbled
1 handful fresh basil, chopped
1 spring onion (scallion), finely chopped
2 teaspoons groundnut oil

SERVES 2

Method

Grate the courgette, then using a tea towel, or your hand, squeeze all the liquid from it. In a large bowl, mash the butterbeans, basil, spring onion, courgette and feta. Combine them together well. Divide the mixture and using your hand, mould it into little patties. Place in the fridge for 10 minutes to firm up. Coat a frying pan with oil and cook the patties on either side for around a minute. Remove them to a baking sheet and bake in the oven for 10 minutes 220C/425F. Serve with a green salad and hummus dip.

DINNER

Most of us find it easier to put together a healthy meal when we have the time but what can make life a lot easier is making too much; leftovers are a good thing. A quick warm up meal the next day or stored in the freezer can be invaluable for throwing together a quick meal, by stirring up leftover meat and veggies in a pan with beaten eggs and making a scramble can be really satisfying.

For all the recipes in this book, avoid fat-free alternatives in yogurt, coconut milk and always use butter instead of margarine. Many of the recipes are low in carbohydrate. To keep your carbohydrate intake down, we've substituted some mashed potatoes for vegetable alternatives like celeriac or sweet potato mash. A lower carbohydrate intake will help reduce cravings for stodgy food and sugar, not to mention boost your vitality and help trim down your waistline. If you want to take it a step further, you can replace the carbohydrate part of your meals with heaps of veggies instead – it won't leave you feeling sluggish.

Chicken & Chorizo Chilli

Ingredients

1 tablespoon olive oil
1 large onion, finely chopped
2 teaspoons chilli power
2 teaspoons cumin
2 x 400g (2x 14oz) cans of
peeled plum tomatoes
475ml (1 pint) chicken stock
225g (8oz) chorizo, diced
4 chicken breasts, sliced
1 red pepper, finely chopped
300g (11oz) can of kidney beans

SERVES 4-6

Method

Warm the oil in a frying pan, add the onion and cook until soft. Add the chilli, cumin and stir. Pour in the tomatoes. Add the stock and bring to the boil. Add the red pepper, chorizo and sliced chicken breasts. Stir and cover. Reduce the heat and simmer for around 15 minutes. Add the kidney beans and simmer for a further 20 minutes.

Instead of serving with rice, you could go for a low carb option and spoon the chicken chilli into iceberg or romaine lettuce leaves to wrap around. Add guacamole and cheese, for a real mouth watering meal which won't leave you feeling heavy.

Sausage & Butternut Squash Mash

SERVES 4

Ingredients

1 butternut squash, peeled and chopped

2 sweet potatoes, peeled and chopped.

8 top-quality sausages

2 apples, cored, peeled and cut into wedges

1/4 teaspoon ground cinnamon

2 teaspoons butter

2 tablespoons wholegrain mustard

1/8 teaspoon ground nutmeg

Method

Coat the sausages with mustard and place them on a baking tray. Sprinkle the apple wedges with cinnamon and add them to the baking tray. Bake in the oven on 200C/400F for 20 to 25 minutes. Meanwhile, add the squash and sweet potatoes to a pan of boiling water. Bring to the boil then reduce the heat. Simmer for around 14 minutes or until tender. Drain the squash and sweet potato, add the butter and ground nutmeg then mash together until soft and smooth. Serve the mash onto plates and add the sausages, apple and cooking juices.

Pork Chops in Pepper Cream Sauce

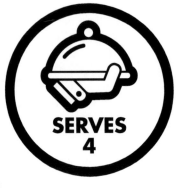

SERVES 4

Ingredients

1 teaspoon coarsely ground black pepper

1/4 teaspoon sea salt

4 boneless pork chops

2 tablespoons olive oil

1 medium shallot, finely chopped

180ml (6fl oz or 3/4 cup) double cream (heavy cream)

Method

Sprinkle the chops with ¼ teaspoon black pepper and ¼ teaspoon salt and pat onto both sides of each pork chop. Heat the oil in a large frying pan over a medium-high heat. Add the chops, reduce the heat and fry for 3 or 4 minutes per side, or until cooked through. Transfer the chops to a plate and cover with foil to keep them warm. Reduce the heat of the frying pan and add the shallot to the pan. Cook for 1 minute, until soft. Pour in the cream and the remaining ¼ teaspoon salt and ¾ teaspoon black pepper and stir until warmed through. Serve the pork chops with the pepper sauce. It goes really well with celeriac mash on the side.

Thai Green Chicken Curry

Ingredients

- 4 chicken breasts, cut into strips
- 50g (2oz) green beans, sliced lengthways
- 4 tablespoons chopped coriander (cilantro)
- 2 stalks of lemon grass (inner stalks), chopped finely
- 400ml coconut milk
- 2 green chillies, chopped and de-seeded
- 2 tablespoons Thai green curry paste
- 1 teaspoon coconut oil
- 4 tablespoons basil leaves, torn,
- 1 tablespoon fish sauce
- Juice of 1 lime

SERVES 4

Method

Heat the coconut oil in a pan and add the green curry paste. Cook for 2-3 minutes. Add the coconut milk and lemongrass and simmer for 5 minutes. Add the chicken, coriander, green beans, and chillies. Bring to the boil and simmer for 15 minutes, uncovered. Add a little boiling water if it seems to be getting dry. Stir in the fish sauce, basil and add the lime juice. Serve with brown rice.

Bacon & Broccoli Hash

SERVES
4

Ingredients

750g (1lb 11oz) sweet potato, peeled and cut into small cubes

200g (7oz) broccoli, cut into small florets

1 tablespoon olive oil

6 slices of bacon, chopped

1 small onion, thinly sliced

Method

In a steamer, cook the sweet potato for 10 minutes. Add the broccoli and cook for another 4 minutes. Heat the oil in a frying pan. Add the bacon and onion. Fry until the bacon is cooked thoroughly and the onion is soft. Add the broccoli and sweet potato to the pan and stir. Cook for around 10 minutes, stirring to dislodge the lovely crispy crust from the bottom.

Barbecue 'Buffalo' Chicken Wings

Ingredients

18 chicken wings
Barbecue sauce:
1 teaspoon cumin
2 teaspoons paprika
1/2 teaspoon cayenne pepper (1 tsp if you like it hot)
1 teaspoon garlic salt
1 teaspoon onion powder
2 tablespoons apple cider vinegar
1 teaspoon pepper
1 teaspoon mustard
1/2 teaspoon stevia (optional)
2 tablespoons olive oil

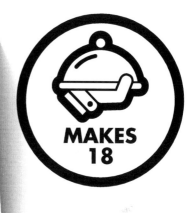

MAKES 18

Method

Preheat the oven to 200C/400F. In a bowl, mix together all the barbecue sauce ingredients and stir really well. Dip the chicken wings in the sauce and place them on a large baking sheet. Place in the oven for 30 minutes, until the chicken wings are cooked through and well browned. Transfer to a serving plate and enjoy.

Chilli & Lime Turkey Strips

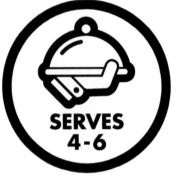

SERVES
4-6

Ingredients

1lb (500g) turkey
2 tablespoons coconut oil
1½ teaspoons chilli powder
2 cloves of garlic, crushed
Juice of 1 lime

Method

Slice the turkey into small strips. Heat the coconut oil in a frying pan over a medium heat and add the turkey. Stir-fry the strips for 2 to 3 minutes, then add the chilli powder, garlic and lime juice. Continue stirring for another 6 or 7 minutes or until cooked thoroughly. These are a great, versatile and tasty addition to many dishes. You can add them to salads, rice, stir fries and wraps. They can also be a handy high protein snack for lunch on the go.

Celeriac Mash

Ingredients
1 celeriac
25g (1oz) butter
Salt & pepper

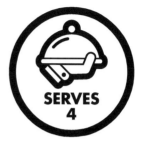

SERVES 4

Method

Peel the celeriac then chop into chunks. Place in a saucepan of cold water. Bring to the boil and simmer for 20 minutes. Drain the celeriac and mash with the butter. Season with salt and pepper.

Sweet Potato Mash with Ginger & Nutmeg

Ingredients

700g (1lb 9 oz) sweet potato, peeled and chopped
1 teaspoon ground ginger,
1/2 teaspoon nutmeg

1/2 teaspoon garlic powder
2 teaspoons butter
Sea salt
Pepper

SERVES 4

Method

Place the sweet potatoes in a saucepan, bring to the boil and simmer for 10 to 12 minutes, until soft. Drain the sweet potatoes but leave them in the saucepan. Add the ginger, nutmeg, garlic and butter to the sweet potatoes and mash them until they become smooth. Season and serve.

Chicken Casserole

Ingredients

4 large chicken legs
(including thigh portion)
475ml / pint chicken
or vegetable stock
4 stalks of celery
2 carrots
1 small onion
2 sage leaves
1 large sprig rosemary
2 tablespoons olive oil
Freshly ground black pepper
1 bay leaf

SERVES 4

Method

Preheat the oven to 170C/325F. Season the chicken pieces with black pepper and place in an oven-proof casserole dish. Roughly chop the carrots, celery and onion and add to the casserole dish. Now add the stock to the chicken and vegetables. Using kitchen string, tie together the sage, rosemary and bay leaves and add to the pot. Cover and place in the oven for 1 hour. Check to make sure the chicken is cooked thoroughly. Remember to remove the bunch of herbs before serving.

Salmon & Dill Burgers

Ingredients

600g (1 ½ lb) boneless salmon fillet
50g (2oz or ½ cup) fresh dill
1 garlic clove
1 egg
1 spring onion

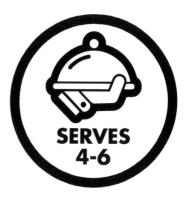

SERVES 4-6

Method

Place the salmon in a food processor with the spring onion, dill and garlic. Blend it until smooth. Place the mixture in a medium bowl and combine with the egg. Using your hands, shape the mixture into patties. Place under a grill for 15 minutes, turning once halfway through.

Salmon & Cod Kebabs with Coriander Pesto

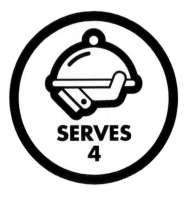

SERVES 4

Ingredients

350g (12oz) piece of cod
350g (12oz) salmon steak
Juice of 1 lime
Freshly ground black pepper to season
Coriander pesto (cilantro pesto)

Method

Remove skin and all bones from both fish. Cut each of them into chunks and place in a bowl. Cover with the lime juice and black pepper. Once the fish is coated, slide alternating pieces of salmon and cod onto metal or wooden skewers. Place the kebabs under a hot grill (broiler) – and cook for 2 to 3 minutes on each side, until cooked through. Serve with coriander pesto (cilantro pesto). See pesto recipe in the sauces and dips section.

Sea Bass Gremolata

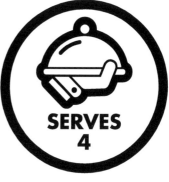

Ingredients

- 4 large sea bass fillets
- 1 lemon
- 1 handful flat-leaf parsley
- 2 cloves of garlic
- 3 tablespoons butter
- 4 handfuls of rocket (arugula)

SERVES 4

Method

Wash the lemon and finely grate the peel to make zest. Chop the parsley and crush the garlic. In a bowl combine the juice and zest from the lemon, parsley and garlic to make the gremolata. Coat the fish fillets. Heat the butter in a frying pan. Add the fish and cook for 3-4 minutes on each side. Spread the gremolata onto the fish, cover the pan with a lid and cook on a low heat for 2 minutes. Serve on a bed of rocket (arugula) and eat immediately.

Parma Ham & Turkey Roll

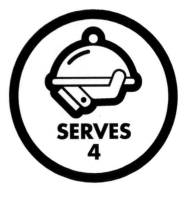

SERVES 4

Ingredients

4 turkey escallops
2 garlic cloves, chopped finely
Juice and grated rind of a lemon
4 slices of Parma ham (alternatively
use any ham or bacon)
2 tablespoons chopped fresh basil
or chives
2 tablespoons olive oil
Salt and pepper

Method

Halve each turkey escalope horizontally and open it out. Season the inside of the turkey with salt and pepper, then sprinkle with garlic, lemon juice, lemon rind and chopped herbs. Put the two pieces back together again. Wrap the turkey in a slice of ham and hold it together with wooden cocktail sticks. Heat the olive oil in a frying pan. Add the turkey rolls and cook for 4-5 minutes until they are golden brown. Turn over, and coat with any remaining lemon juice. Cook for another 3-4 minutes until cooked through then serve.

Turkey Burgers

Ingredients

1lb (500g) minced turkey
1 small onion, finely chopped
½ teaspoon Tabasco sauce
1 teaspoon dried thyme
1 beaten egg
1 tablespoon olive oil

SERVES 4

Method

Add all the ingredients to a bowl, stir and combine. Divide the mixture into 8. Mould into patty shapes and flatten. In a large frying pan, heat the olive oil. Add the burgers and cook for 4-5 minutes on each side until cooked through and golden.

Paprika & Garlic Oven Roast Chicken

SERVES 4-6

Ingredients

1 large whole chicken
1 tablespoon olive oil
1 teaspoon paprika
1 teaspoon garlic salt
Freshly ground black pepper
Sea salt

Method

Preheat your oven to 220C/425F. Place the olive oil, paprika and garlic into a small bowl and stir. Place the chicken in an oven-proof dish. Rub the mixture over the whole chicken, making sure it's completely covered. Sprinkle with salt and freshly ground black pepper. Place in the oven and cook for around 1 hour 15 minutes or until the chicken juices run clear. Remove from the oven, cover with foil and allow it to stand for a few minutes before serving.

Coriander & Lime Chicken Skewers

SERVES 4

Ingredients

2 tablespoons olive oil

60ml (2fl oz or 1/4 cup) soy sauce

1/2 teaspoon Tabasco sauce

2 cloves garlic, minced

3 tablespoons chopped fresh coriander (cilantro)

2 small limes, juiced

4 chicken breasts, cubed

1 red pepper (Bell pepper), sliced

1 onion, cut into eighths

Method

In a large bowl, mix together the olive oil, soy sauce, Tabasco, garlic, coriander and lime. Add the chicken and stir. Place in the refrigerator for 2 hours. When you're ready, thread alternating pieces of chicken, peppers, and onion onto skewers. Place under a hot grill (broiler) until the chicken is fully cooked, about 10 to 15 minutes.

Thyme & Lemon Chicken

SERVES 6

Ingredients

9 00g (2lb) chicken thighs
10 sprigs of fresh thyme
250ml (8fl oz or 1 cup) vegetable stock
4 lemons
Salt and pepper

Method

Preheat the oven to 180C/350F. Take the leaves from 5 of the sprigs of thyme and place them between the chicken skin and the meat. Place in an oven-proof dish and season with salt and pepper. Pour in the stock. Quarter the lemons and add them to the dish. Add the remaining thyme sprigs. Place the chicken in the oven and roast for 30 – 40 minutes, or until the chicken is cooked thoroughly.

Pesto Pork with Mozzarella & Tomato

SERVES 4

Ingredients

- 1 tablespoon pitted green olives
- 1 tablespoon pitted black olives
- 300g (11oz) mozzarella cheese
- 2 tomatoes
- 4 pork boneless cutlets
- 5 tablespoons olive oil
- 4 tablespoons basil pesto
- Fresh basil leaves
- Freshly ground black pepper

Method

Preheat the oven to 200C/400F. Slice the tomatoes and olives then set aside. Drain and slice the mozzarella and set aside. Heat 1 tablespoon of olive oil in a frying pan and sear the cutlets for around 30 seconds on either side. Put the remaining oil in an oven-proof dish and add the pork cutlets. Spread a teaspoon of pesto onto each cutlet. Sprinkle them with sliced olives. Add the sliced tomatoes and mozzarella. Bake for 12-15 minutes. Serve and garnish with a few basil leaves.

Mediterranean Herb Quinoa

Ingredients

200g (7oz) quinoa, cooked
2 cloves garlic, crushed
60ml (2fl oz or 1/4 cup) olive oil
Juice of 2 lemons
1/4 teaspoon sea salt
1/4 teaspoon freshly ground black pepper
6 spring onions, (scallions), finely chopped
8 cherry tomatoes, quartered
1/2 cucumber, cubed
2 tablespoons fresh mint, finely chopped
2 tablespoons fresh coriander, (cilantro), finely chopped
1 handful fresh parsley, finely chopped
1 handful rocket (arugula), finely chopped
8 pitted olives, finely chopped
25g (1oz or 1/4 cup) crumbled feta cheese

SERVES 2

Method

In a large bowl, mix together the garlic, olive oil, lemon juice, salt, and pepper. Add the quinoa, spring onions, tomatoes, cucumber, olives, rocket, herbs, and feta cheese. Toss in the dressing until it's well combined. Chill in the fridge for at least 30 minutes before serving for the flavours to infuse.

Spicy Lamb Stew

Ingredients

700g (1 ½ lb) boneless lamb, cut into cubes
2 tablespoons coconut oil
1 large onion, chopped
2 cloves garlic, chopped
1 tablespoon fresh ginger, chopped finely
1 teaspoon cumin
1 teaspoon ground coriander (cilantro)
1 teaspoon ground cinnamon
¼ teaspoon chilli flakes (or more if required)
¼ teaspoon ground cloves
½ cup natural (unflavoured) yogurt
1 tomato, chopped
120 ml (4 fl oz or ½ cup) chicken or vegetable stock
4 tablespoons fresh coriander (cilantro)
Sea salt to season

SERVES 4-6

Method

In a large saucepan, heat the coconut oil. Add the lamb in batches, browning on all sides. Reduce the heat and add in the onion, garlic, cumin, cinnamon, cloves, ginger, salt, chilli and coriander (cilantro). Cook for 2 minutes until the onion begins to soften. Add the yogurt. Stir for a minute or so, until thickened. Add the lamb, tomato and stock and bring to boil. Reduce heat and simmer for 45 minutes. Sprinkle with a little coriander or parsley and serve.

Lamb Curry with Cinnamon & Star Anise

Ingredients

6 garlic cloves, crushed

4 tablespoons coconut oil

1 tablespoon freshly grated ginger, finely chopped

2.5cm (1 inch) cinnamon

2 bay leaves

800g (1lb 12oz) lamb shoulder, cut into cubes

2 onions,

2 star anise

2 teaspoons cumin

1/2 teaspoon cayenne pepper

1 tablespoon paprika

1 tablespoon tomato paste

180ml (6fl oz or 3/4 cup) coconut milk

240ml (8fl oz or 1 cup) chicken or vegetable stock

Method

Heat half the coconut oil in a large frying pan and briefly sauté the garlic and ginger then add the cinnamon and bay leaves. Add the lamb and cook for 5 minutes, browning it on all sides. Place the meat in a bowl and set aside. Heat the remaining oil in the frying pan and add the onions, star anise, cumin, cayenne pepper, paprika and tomato paste. Cook for 2 minutes. Return the meat to the pan. Add the coconut milk and stock then bring to the boil. Reduce the heat and gently simmer for 1 hour, stirring occasionally. After 30 minutes, add a little water if necessary. When the meat is tender it's ready to serve.

Mildy Spiced Chicken Skewers

Ingredients

2 teaspoons turmeric
1/2 teaspoon chilli powder
4 tablespoons lemon juice
2 garlic clove, peeled and crushed
100ml (4fl oz or 1/2 cup) natural
(unflavoured) yogurt
4 chicken breasts, cut into chunks

Method

In a large bowl, mix together the turmeric, chilli powder, lemon juice, garlic and yogurt. Add the chicken and coat thoroughly in the mixture. Thread the chicken pieces onto the skewers. Pour over some of the remaining yogurt mixture. Place under a hot grill (broiler) for 15 minutes, turning occasionally, until the chicken is fully cooked.

Fried Rice & Pork

Ingredients

- 150g (5oz) pork cut into small cubes
- 2 eggs, beaten
- 225g (8oz) mushrooms, chopped
- 350g (12oz or 2 cups) rice, cooked
- 2 tablespoons soy sauce
- 2 spring onions (scallions)
- 3 teaspoons olive oil (or nut oil)
- 2 cloves garlic, crushed

SERVES 2

Method

In a frying pan, heat a teaspoon olive oil, add the spring onions (scallions), and garlic and cook until they become soft. Transfer to a bowl and set aside. Heat a teaspoon of olive oil in the pan, and fry the eggs until they are firm. Place the eggs in a bowl and leave aside. Heat a teaspoon of olive oil in the frying pan then add the pork, soy sauce, mushrooms and rice. Heat thoroughly. Add the cooked spring onions, garlic and eggs. Combine and serve straight away.

Alternatively try using leftover meat from the fridge, like turkey, chicken or ham and some leftover vegetables too.

95

Quick & Easy Chicken Curry

SERVES 2

Ingredients

1 onion, chopped

1 tablespoon coconut oil

4 teaspoons medium curry powder

1 teaspoon cumin

1/2 teaspoon ginger

1 bay leaf

2 chicken breasts, cut into slices

250ml (8fl oz or 1 cup) chicken stock

1/2 teaspoon salt

1/2 teaspoon pepper

Method

In a frying pan, sauté the onion in oil until it becomes soft. Add the cumin, curry, ginger and the bay leaf and cook for 5 minutes. Add the chicken stock, and chicken. Cook for 10-12 minutes. Season with salt and pepper, if required.

Parmesan Chicken

SERVES 6

Ingredients

6 chicken breasts

100g (3½ oz or 1 cup) grated Parmesan cheese

4 teaspoons garlic powder

1 teaspoon oregano

1 teaspoon paprika

1 teaspoon pepper

2 eggs

2 tablespoons butter

Method

In a bowl, combine the Parmesan cheese with the oregano, garlic, paprika and pepper. In a separate bowl, whisk the eggs. Dip the chicken breasts in the beaten egg, followed by a generous dip in the cheese and herb mixture, making sure you coat both sides really well. Melt the butter in a frying pan over a medium heat. Add the chicken breasts and cook for 4 or 5 minutes on each side, or until cooked through.

Cajun Salmon

Ingredients

2 salmon fillets
1 teaspoon Cajun seasoning
2 cloves of garlic, crushed.
2 tablespoons butter

SERVES 2

Method

The recipe for the seasoning is in the sauces and dips section. Sprinkle the skinless side of the salmon with the Cajun seasoning. Melt the butter in a frying pan over a medium heat, and add the salmon, skin side down. Cook for 4 to 5 minutes on each side, turning gently. Remove and place the salmon fillets onto a serving plate. Stir the garlic into the butter remaining in the pan. Cook for 2 minutes or so, then pour all the garlic butter over the salmon and serve.

Thai Vegetables

Ingredients

2 tablespoons coconut oil

1 onion, sliced

650g (1lb 7oz) mixed vegetables, celery, green beans, carrots, broccoli, chopped

2-3 teaspoons thai red curry paste

350ml (12fl oz) boiling water

200ml (7fl oz) coconut milk

1 tablespoon fresh coriander leaves (cilantro), chopped

50g (2oz) chopped peanuts, to garnish

SERVES 4-6

Method

Heat the coconut oil in a large pan. Add the onion and cook for 3-4 minutes. If you are using carrots, add them first and fry for 2 minutes. Add the remaining vegetables and cook for a further 2 minutes. Add the curry paste and the boiling water. Cover and simmer for 10 minutes until the vegetables are tender but firm. Stir in the coconut milk and add the coriander (cilantro). Heat through. Transfer to serving bowls and scatter with chopped peanuts.

Chicken & Avocado Salad

Ingredients

1 cup black eyed peas
2 skinless cooked chicken breast, shredded
½ cucumber, peeled, deseeded and chopped
1 avocado, flesh scooped out
Dash of Tabasco sauce
Juice of ½ lemon
2 teaspoons olive oil
6 Little Gem lettuce leaves
1 teaspoon mixed seeds (sunflower, sesame or flaxseed)

SERVES 2

Method

Rinse the black-eyed peas in cold water and drain. Put the chicken, peas and cucumber in a bowl. Place the avocado, Tabasco, lemon juice and olive oil in a food processor and blitz until smooth. Combine the avocado mixture with the chicken and black eyed peas. Spoon the mixture into the lettuce leaves. Sprinkle with the seeds. Chill and serve.

Vegetarian Chilli

SERVES
2

Ingredients

- 1 small onion, chopped finely
- 150g (5 ½ oz) kidney beans
- 2 cloves garlic, crushed
- 2 teaspoons olive oil
- ½ teaspoon ground cumin
- 125g (4 ½ oz) mushrooms, finely chopped
- 1 small aubergine, finely diced
- 1 tablespoon tomato paste
- 120ml (4fl oz or ½ cup) vegetable stock
- 1 teaspoon chilli powder (or 2 if you like it hot)
- 1 teaspoon dried mixed herbs

Method

In a large saucepan, heat the olive oil. Add the onion and garlic and soften slightly. Add the mushrooms, aubergines, tomato paste, vegetable stock, chilli, cumin and mixed herbs. Bring to the boil then simmer for 30 minutes, stirring occasionally. Add the kidney beans and cook for another 10 minutes. Serve with rice, or go carbohydrate free and scoop the chilli into lettuce leaves. Iceberg or romaine lettuce work best. It's even better topped with grated cheese and guacamole – you won't miss the carbs!

Pork Chops, Mushrooms & Sour Cream

SERVES 6

Ingredients

6 pork chops
1 onion, sliced
200g mushrooms, sliced
475ml (1 pint or 2 cups) chicken stock
240ml (8fl oz or 1 cup) sour cream
(or crème fraiche)
1 teaspoon olive oil
Garlic powder
Sea salt
Freshly ground black pepper

Method

Season pork chops with salt, pepper and garlic powder. In a frying pan, heat the olive oil and lightly brown the chops. Place them in a slow cooker and top with slices of mushroom and onion. Pour the chicken stock over the chops. Cover and cook on low for 7 to 8 hours. Season with salt and pepper. When you are ready to serve, pour the meat juices into a saucepan, add the sour cream and heat through, stirring continuously. Serve the chops and pour over the sauce.

Chilli Beef & Broccoli

Ingredients

1 tablespoon ground nut oil
100g (3 ½ oz or 3/4 cup) broccoli, broken into florets
300g (11 oz) beef, thinly sliced
5cm piece fresh ginger, peeled and finely chopped
2 cloves garlic, chopped
½ red chilli, deseeded and finely chopped
125ml (4fl oz or ½ cup) water
2 spring onions (scallions) finely chopped

SERVES 2

Method

In a wok or pan warm the oil over a high heat. Put the broccoli, garlic, ginger and chilli into the pan. Stir and cook for 2 minutes. Add the sliced beef and water. Bring to the boil and keep on a high heat for 2 minutes. Add the spring onions and cook for another minute. Serve into bowls and eat immediately.

Braised Beef
& Chestnut Mushrooms

Ingredients

1.35kg (2lb) braising steak (chuck steak), thickly sliced

2 onions, thinly sliced

2 tablespoons dried porcini mushrooms

3 tablespoons olive oil

1 tablespoon plain (all purpose) flour

250g (9 oz) chestnut mushrooms, halved

Sea salt

Freshly ground black pepper

**SERVES
8**

Method

Pour 600ml boiling water over the dried mushrooms. Soak for 30 minutes, then drain, reserving the juices. Season the beef on both sides with salt and pepper. Heat 2 tablespoons of olive oil in a pan, then add the meat and cook until browned. Remove the meat from the pan and set aside. Add to the pan 1 tablespoon of olive oil, then add the onions and fry until softened. Return the meat to the pan, sprinkle in the flour and cook for 1 min. Place the onions and meat in an oven-proof casserole dish and add the mushroom liquid and soaked mushrooms. Season and cover. Cook in the oven for 1½-2 hours at 150C/300F until the meat is tender. After an hour, add the chestnut mushrooms and stir then leave to continue cooking. Serve with celeriac mash.

Blue Cheese Burgers

Ingredients

40g (1 ½ oz) blue cheese
250g (9 oz) lean minced beef
(ground beef)
2 tablespoons fresh parsley,
finely chopped
Freshly ground black pepper
1 tablespoon groundnut oil

SERVES 2

Method

In a bowl, break the cheese and roll it into 4 balls. In a large bowl, mix the beef, parsley and black pepper then divide the mixture into 4. Roll into small balls. Make a deep well in the middle of each ball and place the cheese inside it. Cover with meat and seal it so that no cheese is visible inside and flatten it slightly. Repeat for the other beef balls. Heat the oil in a frying pan over a high heat. Add the burgers and quickly brown for about 1 minute on each side. Reduce the heat and cook for around 3 minutes on each side. This lends itself well to other types of cheeses too, if blue cheese isn't for you.

Thai Beef

Ingredients

2 tablespoons groundnut oil
300g (11 oz) beef strips, or steak cut into thin strips
1 red chilli, deseeded and finely sliced
1 clove garlic, crushed
2 tablespoons soy sauce
2 tablespoons fresh basil leaves, chopped

SERVES 2

Method

Heat the oil in a wok or large frying pan. Add the beef strips, garlic and chilli. Stir and cook for 2-3 minutes or until the meat is lightly browned. Add the soy sauce. Cook until heated through. Stir in the basil leaves. Serve with rice and salad.

Coconut Dahl

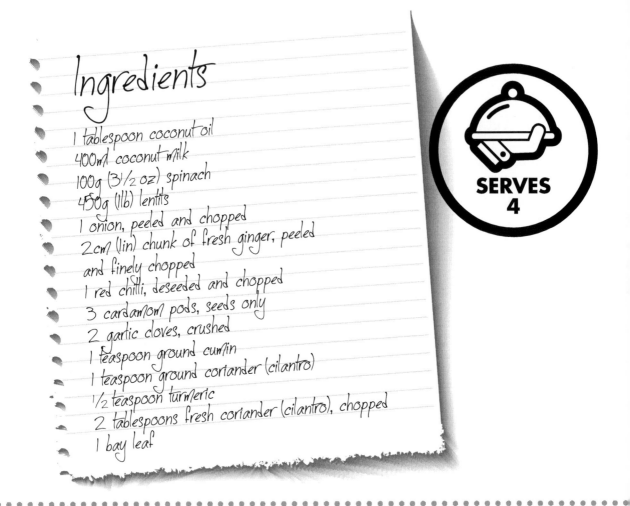

Ingredients

1 tablespoon coconut oil
400ml coconut milk
100g (3½ oz) spinach
450g (1lb) lentils
1 onion, peeled and chopped
2cm (1in) chunk of fresh ginger, peeled and finely chopped
1 red chilli, deseeded and chopped
3 cardamom pods, seeds only
2 garlic cloves, crushed
1 teaspoon ground cumin
1 teaspoon ground coriander (cilantro)
½ teaspoon turmeric
2 tablespoons fresh coriander (cilantro), chopped
1 bay leaf

SERVES 4

Method

Heat the coconut oil in a large saucepan. Add the onion, ginger, cumin, ground coriander, turmeric, cardamom seeds, chilli and garlic and cook for about 10 minutes or until the onion is soft. Add the lentils, coconut milk and bay leaf. Cook for 15 minutes. Add the spinach and stir. Cook for another 3 minutes. Just before serving, add the fresh coriander and stir in. Serve with salad or brown rice.

DESSERTS, SWEET TREATS & SNACKS

If you have a sweet tooth then this may be the section you've skipped to. As well as dessert recipes we have included snack options to give you something to nibble on in between meals or for a case of the after dinner munchies when you raid the cupboards thinking 'what can I eat'. Our chocolate recipes contain 100% cocoa powder and stevia as a sweetener giving you the fabulous chocolate hit but keeping it sugar-free. But a note of caution, we know it can awaken the taste buds to the possibility of other sweet things and it could test your will power against other desserts which aren't sugar free.

Therefore, eat these in moderation occasionally, not instead of a meal. We want you to carry on your new way of eating healthily but we know how important it is to enjoy your food. If you're unsure about testing yourself with sweet things, the temptation is too great, or it's still early days with your sugar-free diet, hold back those cravings by snacking on a selection of cheeses, olives or nuts after a meal and it won't seem like a hardship.

Spicy Mixed Nuts

Ingredients

2 tablespoons coconut oil

80g (½ cup) almonds

80g (½ cup) cashew nuts

80g (½ cup) Brazil nuts

80g (½ cup) macadamia nuts

80g (½ cup) pecan nuts

80g (½ cup) walnuts

½ teaspoon cayenne pepper

½ teaspoon nutmeg

Sprinkling of sea salt

SERVES 6-8

Method

Heat the coconut oil in a large frying pan. Add the nuts, cayenne pepper, nutmeg and salt. Stir constantly for around 7-8 minutes. Store or serve as a party nibble or snack. A variation is to substitute the cayenne pepper and nutmeg for curry powder for an extra fiery kick.

Courgette Chips (Zucchini)

SERVES 2

Ingredients

1 large courgette
1 teaspoon olive oil
Sea salt (paprika, cayenne pepper
or garlic powder can be used)

Method

Slice the courgette (zucchini) into thin circles, around the thickness of a coin. Place them in a bowl, add a teaspoon of olive oil and seasoning. Toss to lightly coat them. Line a baking sheet with foil, and lay out the slices onto the sheet. Preheat the oven to 220C/425F and bake the chips 30 minutes, turning once. Remove when crispy and golden. Serve and eat immediately.

Kale Chips

SERVES 4

Ingredients

1 bag of fresh kale
1 tablespoon olive oil
Sea salt and black pepper to season

Method

Remove the stalks from the kale and cut the leaves into bite-size squares, of around 3cms. Put the oil, pepper and salt in a bowl and toss the kale to coat it. Place on a baking tray and cook the kale in the oven at 170C/325F for 6-10 minutes, until crispy.

Cherry & Almond 'Cheesecake'

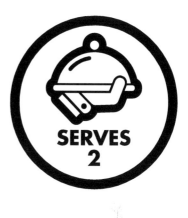

SERVES 2

Ingredients

300g (12oz) cherries, stones removed
200g (8oz) ricotta cheese
50g (2oz) flaked almonds
75g (3oz) ground almonds

Method

Heat the cherries in a saucepan until warmed through. Sprinkle the ground almonds onto the bottom of two serving bowls. Spoon the ricotta cheese on top. Pour the warm cherries over the ricotta. Sprinkle with flaked almonds. Eat immediately.

Spiced Pears with Mascarpone

SERVES 4

Ingredients

200g (7oz) mascarpone
4 large ripe Conference pears
75g (3oz) butter
1 cinnamon stick, snapped into pieces
8 cloves
1 teaspoon orange rind
2 star anise

Method

Peel the pears and trim the bottom slightly to allow them to stand up. Heat the butter in a frying pan, add the cinnamon, cloves and star anise. Once the butter is warm, add the pears. Gently cook for 10-15 minutes, basting the pears with the butter and spice. Combine the mascarpone with the orange rind in a bowl and set aside. When the pears are soft and cooked through, transfer into bowls and serve with a side dollop of mascarpone.

Coconut Snack Bars

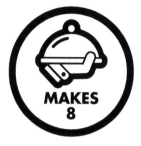

MAKES 8

Ingredients
- 100g (4oz or 1 cup) desiccated coconut (shredded)
- 2 tablespoons coconut oil
- 1/2 teaspoon vanilla extract
- 1-2 teaspoons stevia powder
- Pinch of salt (1/8 tsp)

Method

Place all the ingredients into a food processor. Scrape out the coconut mixture into the bottom of a loaf tin or small rectangular container. Spread and smooth the mixture. Chill in the fridge for one hour. Cut into 8 slices and keep chilled until you're ready to serve.

Banana Chocolate Bites

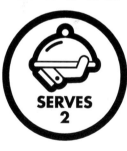

SERVES 2

Ingredients
- 4 teaspoons cocoa powder
- 4 teaspoons desiccated coconut
- 2 bananas, sliced diagonally

Method

Put the cocoa powder and coconut on separate plates. Roll each banana slice in the cocoa, shake off the excess and dip into the coconut. Set on a plate and eat immediately.

Chocolate Brazil Nut Brittle

Ingredients

150g Brazil nuts, chopped
75g (3oz) coconut oil
75g (3oz) butter
2 tablespoons 100% cocoa powder
or raw cacao powder
2 teaspoons stevia powder

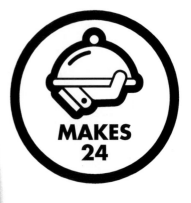

MAKES 24

Method

Melt the butter and coconut oil in a saucepan. Stir in the cocoa powder and stevia and stir until smooth. Place half of the chopped Brazil nuts in the bottom of a small dish or small loaf tin. Pour onto half the chocolate mixture. Sprinkle on the remaining chopped nuts and add the remaining chocolate. Chill for at least an hour until the chocolate has hardened. Using a knife, cut into 24 small pieces or break into rough chunks and serve. The coconut oil will melt in a warm room so it needs to be kept chilled until ready to eat. As a variation, try adding chopped banana with the Brazil nuts before covering with chocolate. It's so delicious.

Nut Butter Chocolates

Ingredients

75g (3oz) coconut oil
75g (3oz) butter
2 tablespoons 100% cocoa powder
or raw cacao powder
2 teaspoons stevia powder
Jar of peanut, almond, cashew
or pistachio butter

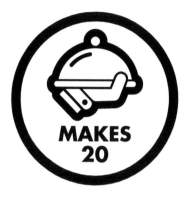

MAKES 20

Method

Place the coconut oil, butter, cocoa powder and stevia powder into a saucepan and heat until the butter and coconut oil have melted and the mixture is smooth. Set out small paper cake cases, petit four size works best. Spoon half the chocolate mixture into the bottom of the paper cases. Only fill each case half way up. Allow to cool slightly. Add 1 teaspoon of nut butter to each case. You may need to re-heat the chocolate if it's beginning to set. Spoon the remaining chocolate into the cases to completely cover the nut butter. Place in the fridge to set for at least an hour.

Raspberry, Lime & Coconut Fool

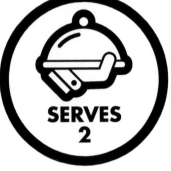

SERVES 2

Ingredients

100g (3 ½ oz) plain (unflavoured) yogurt

1 tablespoon toasted coconut flakes

100g (3 ½ oz) raspberries

Zest and juice of ½ a lime

1 passion fruit

Method

Place the raspberries in a blender and puree until smooth. Put the yogurt, lime zest and juice in a bowl and stir. Add in the raspberry puree, but don't mix it completely, aim for a swirled affect. Spoon the yogurt and raspberry mixture into 2 serving glasses or bowls. Top it with the passion fruit seeds and toasted coconut flakes.

Berry Ice-Cream Popsicles

Ingredients

150g (5 ½ oz or 1 cup)
raspberries or blueberries
350ml (12 fl oz or 1 ½ cups)
plain yogurt (unflavoured)

SERVES 4

Method

Set aside a few of the berries to add whole to the popsicles. Blitz the remaining berries in a food processor until smooth. Add the yogurt to the berries, stirring slowly to achieve a swirly effect. Stir in the remaining whole berries. Spoon the mixture into the ice-lolly moulds. Pop a few berries in as you fill the moulds. Transfer them to the freezer for at least 2 hours until they are frozen solid. For variety, try different combinations of fruit. You can even also add a little fresh herb like basil. Strawberries and mint are a great combination.

Cardamom, Bananas & Vanilla Yogurt

SERVES 2

Ingredients

- 2 tablespoons plain (unflavoured) yogurt
- 1 vanilla pod
- 3 teaspoons coconut oil
- 2 bananas, peeled and halved lengthways
- 2 cardamom pods, seeds removed and crushed
- 2 tablespoons flaked almonds
- Zest and juice of 1 lime

Method

Place the yogurt into a bowl, scrape out the vanilla seeds and stir them in. Set aside. Heat 1 teaspoon of coconut oil in a frying pan. Add the bananas and cook for about 2 minutes on each side until golden. Put the bananas in 2 serving dishes. Using the same pan, heat two teaspoons of coconut oil. Add the crushed cardamom seeds, and flaked almonds and heat for around a minute. Add in the lime juice and zest. Stir until it begins to bubble. Pour the sauce over the bananas. Spoon the yogurt alongside the bananas. Serve and eat straight away.

Raspberry & Chocolate Ice Cream

SERVES 4

Ingredients

225g (8oz or 1 1/3 cups) raspberries
950ml (2 pints or 4 cups) plain yogurt, (unflavoured)
2 tablespoons 100% cocoa powder
Raspberries to garnish

Method

Place the raspberries in a bowl and mash with a fork. Add ½ the yogurt and stir until combined. In another bowl, combine the remaining yogurt and cocoa powder. Line a small loaf tin with grease-proof paper or plastic wrap. Spread ½ the raspberry yogurt mixture into the prepared tin and smooth it. Top it with the chocolate yogurt mixture then add the remaining raspberry mixture. Freeze for at least 3 hours, or until firm. Place a serving plate over the tin and gently tip out the frozen dessert. Remove the wrap. Garnish with a few fresh raspberries, slice and serve.

Yogurt Toppers

Yogurt is so versatile and can be eaten as a snack, breakfast or after a meal. You can liven up your plain yogurt to make it feel like more of a treat. Here are a few suggestions.

COCONUT & PISTACHIO

Chop a tablespoon of toasted coconut flakes and a tablespoon of pistachio nuts. Sprinkle them onto your bowl of yogurt for extra flavour and crunch.

CHOCOLATE, BANANA & BRAZIL NUTS

Cut the banana into diagonal slices, roughly chop the Brazil nuts and add both to your yogurt. Sprinkle with a few raw cacao nibs or cocoa powder and enjoy.

BLUEBERRIES & FLAKED ALMOND

Place a handful of blueberries in a pan, add a pinch of cinnamon and add a squeeze of lemon juice. Pour the warm blueberries over your bowl of yogurt and top if off with flaked almonds.

SAUCES AND DIPS

Guacamole

Ingredients

2 ripe avocados
1 clove garlic
1 red chilli pepper, finely chopped
Juice of 1 lime
2 tablespoons fresh coriander leaves
(cilantro), chopped

Method

Remove the stone from the avocado and scoop out the flesh. Combine all the ingredients in a bowl and mash together until smooth. Garnish with fresh coriander.

Hummus

Ingredients

2 cloves garlic
240g (8oz) can of chickpeas, drained
1 teaspoon sea salt
Juice of 2 lemons
1 tablespoon olive oil

Method

Place all the ingredients in a blender until it is combined. Transfer the hummus into a bowl and it's ready to serve.

Barbecue Sauce

Ingredients

1 teaspoon cumin
2 teaspoons paprika
1/2 teaspoon cayenne pepper
1 teaspoon garlic salt
1 teaspoon cinnamon
2 tablespoons apple cider vinegar
1 teaspoon pepper
1 teaspoon mustard
1/2 teaspoon stevia (optional)
2 tablespoons olive oil

Method

Stir all of the ingredients together in a small bowl and mix well. Store in a container or use it straight away. It works great with chicken wings, ribs, pork or beef.

This barbecue sauce can be used as a marinade for meat before cooking or simply rub it on just before you need it.

Sugar-Free Ketchup

Ingredients

170ml (6oz) tomato paste

2 tablespoons of onion powder

1 teaspoon garlic powder

1/2 teaspoon ground sea salt

150ml (5fl oz) apple cider vinegar

60ml (2fl oz) water

1/8 teaspoon of ground cloves

1/8 teaspoon cinnamon

1/8 teaspoon allspice

1/8 teaspoon pepper

Method

Place all the ingredients in a bowl and stir until smooth. Keep the ketchup in a glass jar in the refrigerator, ready to use.

Coriander Pesto (Cilantro)

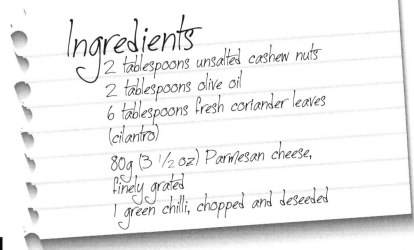

Ingredients

2 tablespoons unsalted cashew nuts
2 tablespoons olive oil
6 tablespoons fresh coriander leaves (cilantro)
80g (3 ½ oz) Parmesan cheese, finely grated
1 green chilli, chopped and deseeded

Method

Place all the ingredients in a food processor and blitz until it becomes a smooth paste.

Basil Pesto

Ingredients

4 tablespoons pine nuts
6 tablespoons basil leaves
80g (3 ½ oz) Parmesan cheese, finely grated
1 clove of garlic
2 tablespoons olive oil

Method

Put all of the ingredients into a food processor or blend until you have a smooth paste.

Mint Pesto

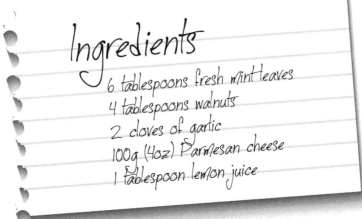

Ingredients

- 6 tablespoons fresh mint leaves
- 4 tablespoons walnuts
- 2 cloves of garlic
- 100g (4oz) Parmesan cheese
- 1 tablespoon lemon juice

Method

Put all the ingredients into a food processor and blend until it becomes a smooth paste.

Cajun Seasoning

Ingredients

- 2½ tablespoons paprika
- 2 tablespoons sea salt
- 2 tablespoons garlic powder
- 1 tablespoon onion powder
- 1 tablespoon cayenne pepper
- 1 tablespoon dried oregano
- 1 tablespoon dried thyme

Method

Mix the ingredients together in a bowl, store in an airtight container or jar and add this versatile seasoning to perk-up chicken, seafood, chops and steak.

Classic Vinaigrette

Ingredients
4 tablespoons olive oil
1 tablespoon apple cider vinegar
(or lemon juice)
1/4 teaspoon sea salt
A squeeze of lemon juice
Freshly ground black pepper

Method

Mix the ingredients together in a bowl or shaker before serving and use with fresh salads. With all the following vinaigrette recipes, you could substitute the vinegar for lemon juice, or try other varieties of vinegar instead.

Garlic Vinaigrette

Ingredients
4 tablespoons olive oil
1 tablespoon apple cider vinegar
1 clove garlic, crushed
A squeeze of lemon juice
1/4 teaspoon salt
Freshly ground black pepper

Method

Mix all the ingredients together and store or use straight away.

Walnut Vinaigrette

Ingredients

4 tablespoons walnut oil
2-3 tablespoons apple cider vinegar
Freshly ground black pepper

Method

Stir the ingredients together and season with sea salt. Can be stored in the fridge or used immediately.